"*Healthy Embodiment* is rich and timely contribution to the phenomenology of embodiment and the philosophy of health and illness. By focusing specifically on the meaning and experience of health, Bas de Boer offers an astute Foucauldian critique that illuminates the extent to which technologies of biomedicine and public health policies discipline the body and shape our understanding and experience of health. The book will be a valuable resource in the philosophy of medicine and critical health studies for years to come."

—**Kevin Aho**, *Florida Gulf Coast University, USA*

Healthy Embodiment

This book provides a philosophical analysis of the experience of health and investigates how this experience is shaped by recent developments in medicine and public health. It shows how phenomenological and Foucauldian approaches to health can be systematically integrated into a general account of healthy embodiment.

Many medical practitioners argue for a shift from curative to preventative medicine. Technoscientific developments now enable us to track our health and provide more effective ways to live healthily. This book argues that these developments shape how we experience our health of and others, as well as the way in which we distinguish between health and illness. Its starting point is that health is not so much an object with well-defined boundaries that can be scrutinised scientifically but is better understood as an embodied experience. The author uses phenomenology and the work of Foucault to develop a theory of healthy embodiment. He argues that experiencing oneself as a healthy subject requires being made present as a healthy object by someone or something else. He explores how the experience of health results from the interaction between being a subject and being an object and potentially involves challenging medical norms.

Healthy Embodiment will be of interest to researchers and graduate students working in phenomenology, science and technology studies, medical humanities, bioethics and sociology of medicine.

Bas de Boer is an assistant professor in the philosophy of technology at the University of Twente. He is the author of *How Scientific Instruments Speak* (2021) and editor of the recent volume *Phenomenology and the Philosophy of Technology* (2024).

Routledge Research in Phenomenology

Edited by Søren Overgaard, *University of Copenhagen, Denmark*, Komarine Romdenh-Romluc, *University of Sheffield, UK*, and David Cerbone, *West Virginia University, USA*

Towards a Phenomenology of Values
Investigations of Worth
D.J. Hobbs

Mechanisms and Consciousness
Integrating Phenomenology with Cognitive Science
Maren Pokropski

Phenomenology as Critique
Why Method Matters
Edited by Andreea Smaranda Aldea, David Carr, and Sara Heinämaa

Contemporary Phenomenologies of Normativity
Norms, Goals, and Values
Edited by Sara Heinämaa, Mirja Hartimo, and Ilpo Hirvonen

Merleau-Ponty and Contemporary Philosophy of Perception
Peter Antich

Sartre and Analytic Philosophy
Edited by Talia Morag

Phenomenology of Broken Habits
Philosophical and Psychological Perspectives on Habitual Action
Edited by Line Ryberg Ingerslev and Karl Mertens

The Phenomenology of the Second-Person Plural
Sarah Pawlett Jackson

Healthy Embodiment
Philosophical Reflections on the Experience of Health
Bas de Boer

For more information about this series, please visit: https://www.routledge.com/Routledge-Research-in-Phenomenology/book-series/RRP

Healthy Embodiment

Philosophical Reflections on the Experience of Health

Bas de Boer

Routledge
Taylor & Francis Group
LONDON AND NEW YORK

First published 2025
by Routledge
605 Third Avenue, New York, NY 10158

and by Routledge
4 Park Square, Milton Park, Abingdon, Oxon, OX14 4RN

Routledge is an imprint of the Taylor & Francis Group, an informa business

ISBN: 978-1-032-99114-6 (hbk)
ISBN: 978-1-032-99113-9 (pbk)
ISBN: 978-1-003-60238-5 (ebk)

DOI: 10.4324/9781003602385

Typeset in Sabon
by Deanta Global Publishing Services, Chennai, India

Contents

Acknowledgements

The idea of this book emerged during an interdisciplinary project on using technologies to promote a healthy lifestyle. This project opened my eyes when it came to realising what kinds of decisions underlie designing for a healthy lifestyle and for behaviour change. I especially want to thank Roelof de Vries and Mailin Lemke for their patience when introducing me to the world of designing for health. I also would like to thank Peter-Paul Verbeek for stimulating me to turn my thoughts about the experience of health into a book already at a very early stage.

Some parts of this book are based on (revisions of) material that was published earlier. Permission was obtained to include this material. Chapter 1 contains revised material that was earlier published in "Experiencing objectified health: Turning the body into an object of attention", *Medicine, Healthcare and Philosophy*, *23*(3), 401–411: https://doi.org/10.1007/s11019-020-0994-0. Chapter 3 makes use of material that was earlier published in an article coauthored with Olya Kudina: "Large language models, politics, and the functionalization of language", *AI Ethics:* https://doi.org/10.1007/s43681-024-00564-w. Chapter 4 makes use of material that was earlier published in an article coauthored with Ciano Aydin: "Empowerment: Freud, Canguilhem and Lacan on the ideal of health promotion", *Medicine, Healthcare and Philosophy*, *26*, 301–311. https://doi.org/10.1007/s11019-023-10145-z.

Special thanks to the members of the human–technology relations group at the University of Twente for the stimulating discussions about health and technology, and to Jochem Zwier for his helpful comments on parts of this book. Of course, all mistakes in this book that will be inevitably there, are my own.

Introduction
The Enigma of Health?

In his *The Enigma of Health*, Hans-Georg Gadamer famously points to the enigmatic character of health. On the one hand, being healthy or living a healthy life is an important desire of many people. On the other hand, when asked what health exactly consists in, it is difficult to come up with a precise answer or to name a specific experience. According to Gadamer, this is because "[h]ealth is not a condition that one introspectively feels in oneself. Rather, it is a condition of being involved, of being in the world, of being together with one's fellow human beings, of active and rewarding engagement in one's everyday tasks" (Gadamer, 1996, p. 113). Relatedly, the French physician René Leriche describes health as "life lived in the silence of the organs" (*op. cit.* Canguilhem, 1991, p. 91). Only when we feel ill are we able to say: "I don't feel healthy" but when we do so we have lost the experience that we initially wanted to capture. Experientially, health seems elusive and is not exprience in the course of everyday life (Gadamer, 1996, p. 96).

But is health that elusive? Developments in the biomedical sciences throughout the 20th and 21st centuries are typically described as having enabled a better understanding of health and to have greatly contributed to increasing our lifespan. Moreover, many organisations engage in health promotion activities, and policy documents develop guidelines on how people can become healthier. Must we not concede then, that Gadamer was simply mistaken and that scientific developments have proven that health is not enigmatic at all?

Doing so would, for Gadamer, reveal a misconception of what the enigma of health consists in. Of course, he maintains, it is possible to conceive of health as an object with well-defined boundaries or to attempt to standardise health with reference to certain values. However, such objectifications or standardisations do hardly tell us anything about what health consists in experientially. For him, any technical or scientific approach to health necessarily misses the mark. The main reason for this is that, for Gadamer, medical science is best understood as "the science of illness"

DOI: 10.4324/9781003602385-1

(Gadamer, 1996, p. 105). It is concerned with objectifying and compartmentalising those aspects of one's body that are experienced as threatening and as causing illness. By—for instance—studying pathophysiology, medical scientists are capable of detecting the sources of the ills of patients. However, in doing so, medicine (a) takes the negation of health as its primary object, and (b) implicitly presupposes that health is an object that is to be understood as the sum of those processes that do not give rise to illness.

This is, according to Gadamer, where medicine goes awry: health is not the sum of certain physiological processes and neither can it be inferred from studying illness: "health does not actually present itself to us" (Gadamer, 1996, p. 107) and only manifests in a "general feeling of well-being [through which] we are open to new things, ready to embark on new enterprises and, forgetful of ourselves, scarcely notice the demands and strains which are put on us" (Gadamer, 1996, p. 112). This general feeling resists scientific objectification and neither can be thematised in our experience: it is the transparency that people live through while thematising other aspects of the world.

The goal of this book is to problematise Gadamer's analysis and to suggest that a philosophical analysis of the experience of health is possible. However, this does not necessarily imply to concede that health is indeed an object that is grasped increasingly better by the medical and life sciences. Instead, this book argues that the ways in which health is thematised in the medical and life sciences shape how we experience ourselves as healthy. The problematisation of the alleged enigmatic character of health will take place through the development of an account of the experience of healthy embodiment.

There are three developments that sparked my interest in the phenomenon of healthy embodiment. First, many medical professionals advocate that it is time to transform medicine from a curative into a preventive or personalised endeavour (Prainsack, 2017; Vogt et al., 2016). Gadamer could still note that "the progress of science has been accompanied by a decline in our more general care for health and in preventative medicine in general" (Gadamer, 1996, p. 106). However, many medical practitioners maintain that scientific progress is the avenue towards better healthcare, as it helps transform curative medicine into preventive medicine. A focus on the prevention of diseases with very different origins ranging from genetic dispositions to lifestyle choices should be at the heart of medical practice. Political institutions have developed initiatives to back up this focus on prevention, partly since the population in many Western countries is growing increasingly older, which poses a challenge the (financial) limits of current healthcare infrastructures. For instance, the European Commission promotes and funds the development and use of mobile health technologies that enable people to track aspects of their everyday life that are allegedly relevant to their health. And in the United States, Barack Obama's *Affordable Care Act* promotes the inclusion of preventive services in existing insurance plans.

Second, the focus on prevention, amongst other developments, blurs the boundaries between clinical medicine and public health. The recent COVID-19 pandemic is a case in point: the spread of an infectious disease was in many countries countered with preventive measures ranging from lockdowns to a particular organisation of public space enabling people to maintain a distance from one another. Such measures were taken to prevent people from getting hospitalised and were treated as having a clinical effect. Whereas it is tempting to conceive of the COVID-19 pandemic as an exceptional situation in which our experience of health is shaped by institutional rules and norms, such that the world is organised as a clinic, one of the key messages of this book is that the experience of healthy embodiment is fundamentally dependent on such norms and rules.

Third, technological developments function prominently in the discourse around medical prevention and health promotion. Such technologies range from pacemakers to self-tracking technologies that enable to monitor the aspects of one's daily life (e.g., food intake, physical activity) that are thought to be relevant health parameters. Often, discourses around paradigmatic changes in medicine (e.g., personalised medicine, precision medicine) suggest that the widespread use of such technologies is key to prevention. This is because self-tracking technologies turn previously invisible aspects of our lives into visible objects that can be continuously attended to, which enables people to change these aspects insofar as they are linked to undesirable health outcomes. Our routines, and the flow of everyday life that Gadamer held to be constitutive of health's enigmatic character, then, become visible objects that are part of our field experience. The phenomenologist Alfred Schütz wrote in 1970 that such routine activities are not "within the thematic kernel at all. They remain, to the contrary, in the margin. I may think over my vital practical or theoretical problems while *walking*, *eating*, shaving, *smoking a cigarette*, and so on" (Schütz, 2011, p. 173, my emphasis). The technologies thought to be relevant for preventive medicine reverse this situation and hold the promise of interpreting our routines in terms of our (future) health. The promise of these technologies is precisely to reduce, if not, eliminate the enigmatic character of health by turning it into an observable object.

In light of these developments, this book asks how the experience of healthy embodiment is constituted. More specifically, it investigates the extent to which the objectifying processes that are typical to modern science in general and the biomedical sciences in specific shape our experience of health. Pursuing this issue requires both analysing the constitution of embodiment and understanding how adding the adjective "healthy" refers to a specific constitution of embodiment.

A Naturalistic Approach to Health

It is not self-evident that health should be approached as an embodied experience. One of the central approaches to health takes a naturalistic starting point and argues that health is and should be a value-free concept belonging to the domain of the biomedical sciences. The most prominent naturalistic account of health is Christopher Boorse's biostatistical theory (BST) of health developed in a series of papers in the 1970s. Boorse argued against the idea that health involves some kind of evaluation that is carried out by medical professionals, societal institutions or other relevant actors. In contrast with such positions, which take health to be first and foremost something requiring practical judgement, he holds that "the idea of health ought to be analyzed by reference to physiological medicine alone" (Boorse, 1975, pp. 49–50). Health, then, is viewed as the absence of disease, where "disease" is a physiologically explicable deviation from normal functioning. If, therefore, it can be shown that what constitutes "disease" is something that can be physiologically determined, Boorse holds that it becomes possible to develop a value-free conception of health (i.e., a conception independent of practical judgement).

On Boorse's naturalistic understanding, "health is normal functioning, where the normality is statistical and the functions biological" (1977, p. 542). For this definition to be free of any evaluative judgements, Boorse thus has to show that both the determination of a biological function and that of statistical normality are "a matter of natural science, not evaluative decision" (1977, p. 543).[1] Boorse's notion of function is derived from biology and is defined as "nothing but a standard causal contribution to a goal actually pursued by the organism" (Boorse, 1975, p. 57). For this definition to be value-free (and hence naturalistic), there has to be a standard class of goals that organisms are naturally pursuing, such that no discussion concerning what kind of goals are worth pursuing can take place—such a discussion would inevitably involve a value judgement of one kind or another. An organism is, on Boorse's account, an assemblage of systems and sub-systems that each perform a function, such that they together help the organism to achieve the goals necessary for its self-preservation. For example, the heart is goal-directed towards the supply of blood to the rest of the body, or the liver towards filtering the blood coming from digestion. The function of such sub-systems, then, contributes to the organism as a whole that is goal-directed to eating and moving, and on a higher level towards survival and reproduction (Boorse, 1975, p. 57).

The exact sub-goals an organism needs to pursue in order for its survival and reproduction vary per species, making it such that different organisms have different kinds of sub-systems having different functions with a different goal-directedness. For Boorse, it is only these sub-systems of which it can be said that they have a certain function: "Functions are not attributed [...] to the whole organism at all, but only to its parts, and the functions of a part are its causal contributions to empirically given goals. What goals a type of organism in fact pursues, and by what functions it pursues them, can be decided without considering the value of pursuing them" (Boorse 1975, p. 58). The notion of function, then, appears on Boorse's account simply as the mechanisms needed to effectively realise a specific goal, such that impairments in the mechanism will prevent the specific goal from being realised, eventually undermining the organism's higher-level goals of survival and reproduction.

When accepting this account of function to be value-free, the second thing Boorse has to show is that it can be decided without evaluative judgement what is the normal functioning of a given sub-system within a given species (i.e., showing that his account of statistical normality does not make reference to value judgements). Boorse's approach to normality in this regard is statistical, such that statements about the normality of a certain physiological function "are about a trait's *standard* contribution in some population or reference class" (Boorse, 1977, p. 556). An example of a reference class can be a species as a whole, or a smaller group of a certain species which is sufficiently comparable to function as a relevant class. One can take the human species as a population, leaving out varieties in sex, race or age, which would make it such that a certain part (e.g., the elderly) falls outside the standard distribution and can be classified as unhealthy. Alternatively, one can take a certain age group (e.g., 70 to 80) as a reference class to be able to determine whether or not someone can be considered as healthy *relative to* the rest of the population of this age group. For Boorse, the parameters used to decide upon what is an adequate reference class can be determined with the means of natural science alone: accounts of biological functioning have determined relevant physiological differences between sexes, races and age groups, such that these can be used as reference groups without appealing to evaluative judgements (in contrast with reference classes having values already embedded in them, such as the set of "handsome males").

Hence, according to BST, it is possible to develop a concept of health that is value-free (i.e., relies on the science of physiology alone) when relying on a concept of biological function that attributes functions only to sub-systems within the organism that help fulfilling its goals (e.g., survival and reproduction), and when determining the healthiness (or normality) of the working of these sub-systems only involves a statistical comparison with the average working within a certain reference class. Provided that these desiderata are met, the question of whether or not a given individual is healthy simply is an empirical question that can be scientifically investigated, and which does not involve any kind of normative judgement.

Normativism as the Negation of Naturalism

Normativist accounts of health defend the idea that health can never be only a matter of natural science alone but always involves a value judgement in one way or the other. Thus, these are directly opposed to naturalistic theories, such as Boorse's BST. To make the opposition between normativists and naturalists as clear as possible, I will present normativism here as the negation of Boorse's BST. Accordingly, normativism is presented as being committed to the claim that both the concept of statistical normality and the concept of function inevitably involve evaluative judgements, even on a very basic level.

A first challenge to naturalism can be framed in terms of the value-ladenness of the term "function". This challenge can be traced back to George Canguilhem's seminal work *The Normal and the Pathological*. For Canguilhem, a naturalistic (non-normative) theory of health can only be established when there is a continuity between normal and pathological functioning (i.e., only if it is the case that a pathology is only quantitatively different from the normal). He discusses the case of diabetes to challenge this continuity thesis. One of the crucial factors in diabetes is glycemia; the concentration of sugar and glucose in the blood of an organism. Now, for doctors and researchers, a crucial question is which rate of glycemia warrants speaking about a pathology; after all, every organism has a rate of glycemia due to its food intake, making it a crucial question when this rate reaches a certain threshold such that it undermines normal functioning. Now, according to Canguilhem, the only reasonable criterion to be used when qualifying a certain glycemia rate as abnormal in physiology is whether or not it accelerates the death of the organism as a whole (1991, p. 75). Two things can be derived from the choice of this criterion: (1) the difference between normal and pathological functioning can never be merely quantitative, since the difference is grounded in the difference between life and death, which must be qualitative, and (2) judgements concerning pathologies can never be about isolated functional mechanisms, but always apply to the organism as a whole.

Now, *if* diabetes is not only to be understood in terms of how it affects the functioning of sub-systems but concerns the organism as a whole, then "to be sick means that a man really lives another life, even in the biological sense of the word", such that the origin of a disease (i.e., unhealthiness) must be "sought in the experience men have in their relations with the whole of their environment" (Canguilhem, 1991, p. 88). When this is the case, so normativists hold, normative judgements cannot be avoided: the difference between health and disease becomes the difference between *desirable* and *undesirable* experiences, or *good* and *bad* relations with the environment. Therefore, the states of health and disease are qualitatively different relative to judgements made by both individuals themselves and the physicians treating them. For example, whether or not diabetes can be considered a pathology cannot be established with reference to isolated functional mechanisms, but becomes a matter of evaluating whether or not certain dysfunctions lead to undesirable states of affairs for the organism being treated. Denying this aspect of disease for developing a form of mechanical objectivity is, for Canguilhem, fundamentally misguided since it runs counter to the purpose of medicine. Canguilhem puts it clearly and succinctly: "medicine needs an objective pathology, but research which causes its object to vanish is not objective" (Canguilhem, 1991, p. 87).

A second challenge to naturalism concerns the arbitrariness in the choice of a certain reference class and questions whether the choice for age, sex or race as reference classes is indeed something value-free. As Elselijn Kingma argues, the choice of particular reference classes is crucial for BST to be successful, and as stated, Boorse takes it as uncontroversial that the relevant reference classes are age, sex and race. However, were we to use entirely different reference classes, such as "having Down's Syndrome" or "being a long-term heavy alcohol-user", an entirely different account of health and disease would emerge: "one in which Down's syndrome and liver cirrhosis were normal in these reference classes, and therefore health" (Kingma, 2014, p. 601). The only way for Boorse to maintain that sex, age, and race are the only relevant reference classes is by making prior (i.e., non-scientific) assumptions about what are and are not healthy human forms, or by invoking a value judgement through which long-term heavy alcohol users can be ruled out as a relevant reference class beforehand.

What is mainly at stake in the debates between normativists and naturalists can be illustrated with the following example: for a long time, masturbation has been considered as a disease, believed to cause blindness, and was generally disvalued and considered sinful. From a naturalistic perspective, it is clear that this view was mistaken: we currently know that masturbation is not a cause of blindness, and we have no good reasons to believe that masturbation harms the organism in any other way. Hence, masturbation is part of what can be called healthy behaviour, making it such that other judgements in the past can be qualified as wrong. From the point of view of the normativist, however, masturbation actually *was* a disease due to the mere fact that it was disvalued and considered sinful (Kingma, 2014, p. 598). Naturalists treat this as a problem for normativist accounts of health: *if* we cannot dismiss such previous states of affairs as being wrong, we are opening the door for unwanted relativism, making it impossible to unmask doctors that nowadays *do* conceive of masturbation as a disease as quacks.

The above example and my brief exposition of the normativistic and naturalistic positions in philosophical debates about health do not serve as a means to settle the debate, but rather to reveal two relevant underlying presuppositions: (1) if health must indeed be framed as a property of an organism relative to the population it is part of, a *measurement apparatus* capable of identifying the "normal" function of such a population has to be in place, and (2) in one way or another, medical judgements—regardless of them being normative or value-free—potentially have a bearing on the organism on which they are applied (the [non-]sinfulness of masturbating attests to this). Or to put it somewhat stronger, medicine is a practice that is not primarily about irresponsive organisms that might have some objective properties, but instead concerns individuals that are being influenced by judgements regarding their health status.

These two presuppositions suggest that the distinction between a *theory* of health, the *practices* that use health as a classificatory term, and the *experience* of health cannot be maintained: we cannot straightforwardly accept that "illnesses are merely a subclass of diseases, namely, those diseases that have certain normative features reflected in the institution of medical practice" (Boorse, 1975, p. 56). Hence, there might be good reasons to not exclusively conceive of health as a theoretical term used in medical textbooks (cf. Boorse, 1977, p. 551). Instead of using conceptual analyses of the term "health" to make clear the semantics of the concept and its difference with "disease", it is therefore necessary to turn to experience of health and the way this experience is shaped by the practice of medicine.

An additional reason for why the distinction between theories of health and healthcare practices cannot be maintained is that medicine currently is increasingly turned into a *preventive* medicine. On this view, medicine should not be primarily concerned with the treatment of disease and illness, but instead with preventing disease and illness from occurring in the first place, for example by promoting lifestyle change (cf. Boenink, 2009; Vegter, 2018; Vogt, Hofmann, & Getz, 2016). As a consequence, the boundaries between theoretical concerns in biomedical science and the practical concerns of public health become blurred. Inevitably, practical judgements about the desirability of certain lifestyle become part of medicine.

Constructivist Critique

One of the main goals of developing a naturalistic account of health—as carried out by Boorse—was to isolate judgements regarding physiology and pathology from the value judgements involved in therapeutic and clinical settings (cf. Giroux, 2016, p. 12): value-free concepts of health and disease are, on Boorse's account, "bedrock requirement[s] to block the subversion of medicine by political rhetoric or normative eccentricity" (1997, p. 100). One of the reasons why a naturalistic concept of health might be attractive seems to lie precisely in that it potentially cancels out many forms of unjustified medicalisation (Schramme, 2007). However, *if* the distinction between the theory of health and disease and the experience of health collapses, *then* the naturalistic quest to find the means to prevent medicine from becoming infected by sociopolitical influences appears misguided.

One of the possible responses to the dismantling of the theory-practice opposition is to start investigating what kind of moral assumptions, and political, social and economic interests are fed into health-related practices—and leave it open how health is defined theoretically. In the introduction to an edited volume provocatively entitled *Against Health*, Metzl describes the point of departure for such a position as follows: "Health is a desired state, but it is also a prescribed state and an ideological position. [...] [A]ppealing to health allows for a set of moral assumptions that are allowed to fly stealthily under the radar" (2010, p. 2). For example, utterances such as "smoking is bad for your health" turn health into a moral obligation by questioning if smoking is a habit that can be exercised by a "good person"—after all, a person engaging in a habit that is allegedly unhealthy *must be* weak of will! Other examples are the economic interests of app-developing companies for promoting self-tracking applications as being beneficial for one's health, or the political interests when promoting same-sex marriages as the healthy norm. Welsh (2022) has recently framed such cases in terms of a prevailing "good health imperative" in which individuals are made responsible for their own health status, such that taking care of one's health in relation to particular contingent norms becomes a moral duty. In such cases, a particular notion of health is derived from a normative discourse that constitutes what is "normal" or "healthy", and is subsequently universalised and naturalised without justification.

An important inspiration for this perspective on medicine is the work of Michel Foucault, who argued that medicine is interrelated with the interests of states, resulting in an approach to the human body as a site of discipline and control (e.g., Foucault, 1978, 1980). Often, invoking a certain norm as being "the healthy norm" involves reference to a supposedly value-free understanding of health, such that a certain form of normalisation appears as natural. Critical studies of health and medicine, then, often intend to show what kind of *normalisation apparatuses* are in place, what kind of power they exercise on citizens, and what kind(s) of values and interests feed into the particular conceptions of "normal" that are advocated as value-free. By presenting a particular phenomenon as "normal", it becomes possible to develop programmes of action when citizens deviate from this norm, thereby creating a strong pressure on individuals to conform to a particular type of normality. Since an increasing number of individuals eventually *will* conform to a certain norm, so it is postulated, it will appear natural to treat deviating in a different—and potentially violent—manner. Hence, as a normalisation apparatus, medicine appears as an institution of social control that exercises power on citizens, making individuals to conform and/or orient to certain values and norms of behaviour (Lupton, 2012, p. 10). The institution of medicine introduces a particular politics of the body by instantiating specific regimes of control that individuals are necessarily involved in. Exposing the values that are *actually* in place in the normalisation apparatus then serves to question the desirability of the particular apparatus being in place.

While this approach importantly reveals that—as an institution—medicine provides a powerful discourse to normalise behaviour by prioritising certain norms and values over others, it pays less attention to the embodied experience of oneself as being healthy or ill. By rendering the bodies of individuals to be docile, the body is primarily conceived of as a *recipient* of power. However, health is also an experience of concrete individuals that cannot be reduced to institutional norms, albeit being shaped by them. Although institutionalised norms might shape how individuals experience their own body, they do not seem to exhaust health-related experiences *as* experienced by the subject.

Phenomenological Critique

Another substantial critique on naturalistic and normativist theories of health comes from phenomenology and highlights the embodied experience of health. Phenomenologists typically emphasise that scientific medicine offer a limited view on health and illness that threatens to overlook how people experience health and illness. One of the first attempts to explicitly make phenomenology relevant for medical practice was in Heidegger's *Zollikon Seminars,* a series of seminars that Heidegger gave to practising psychotherapists on the invitation of the psychiatrist Medard Boss (Heidegger, 2001). Heidegger attempts to show in the seminars that there are limits to approaching the body as a corporeal thing amongst other corporeal things. This is because ontologically, humans not just *have* a body with a clear spatiotemporal location that can be observed from the outside but *are* a body in the sense that the body is the horizon of a human's being-in-the-world and co-determines what is existentially familiar. This latter aspect is what Heidegger calls a bodying forth that is irreducible to the mechanistic logic of the natural and life sciences.

This idea is still at the heart of contemporary phenomenological approaches to medicine. For instance, Carel holds that medicine intends to develop naturalistic accounts of diseases (i.e., physiological dysfunction), thereby neglecting the experience of illness. Since the latter cannot be addressed through scientific objectification, medicine needs to be augmented with a focus on the lived experience of illness (Carel, 2016, p. 1). Similarly, Svenaeus holds that naturalism is accompanied with an image of health that equates it with the absence of diseases, thereby viewing it exclusively in biomedical terms. He argues that this image of health constitutes "a too narrow approach to the goal of clinical practice [...] [because while] to find diseases and to cure or mitigate them form significant *parts* of this activity, [...] the activity includes much more than that" (Svenaeus, 2001, p. 114). A phenomenology of health, then, should augment a naturalistic approach by articulating this "much more than that".

Crucial for the phenomenological argument that it is impossible to exclusively cast health in naturalistic terms are the interrelated distinctions between subjective (*Leib*) and objective body (*Körper*) that we find in Husserl's work, as well as the distinction between disease and illness that can be derived from it. The objective body refers to the body qua its biology, it is the place in which physiological processes occur that can be analysed objectively by the biomedical sciences. From this perspective, the body is viewed as one of the objects encountered *in* the world. The lived body, on the contrary, refers to the body as experienced by the living being; it is not an object amongst other objects but a medium through which we understand and experience ourselves and our environment. Whereas the objective body can be analysed from a third-person perspective, the lived body can only be experienced from a first-person perspective. The distinction between disease and illness can be derived from the distinction between objective body and lived body; disease is a state of the living body caused by a physiological dysfunction that can be analysed from a third-person perspective, while illness is an experience of the lived body from a first-person perspective.

A central concern of phenomenological approaches to medicine is thus not primarily that medicine normalises, but rather that it is an *objectification apparatus* that tacitly or explicitly eliminates a central aspect (i.e., lived experiences) of health and illness from view. Since health concerns the life of an individual as a whole, phenomenological accounts of health maintain that there is something essential to health that evades scientific investigation. Since medical professionals are trained to exclusively view the human body in objective terms, so it is argued, experiences of health and illness are systematically treated as being irrelevant. Hence, an important goal of phenomenological analyses of health is to carve out a space in medical practice in which the embodied experience of patients can be articulated, such that it is recognised as crucial to developing an adequate understanding of health and illness in medical practice.

What phenomenological critiques of biomedicine importantly point to is that any theory of health presupposes a theory of the body, and that a naturalistic theory of health mistakenly reduces the body to an object that can be viewed in terms of its physiology. In addition, and more fundamentally, so phenomenologists argue, health concerns the subjective experience of the lived body. In neglecting this, biomedicine fails to come to terms with one of the central aspects of health. In stressing the importance of the lived body for the experience of health, phenomenologists often tend to juxtapose *Leib* and *Körper,* and prioritise the former over the latter. However, *Leib* and *Körper* are not fundamentally different things, but different *aspects* of the same body that point to the possibility of different *experiences of* and *perspectives on* the body; after all, one's body always also *is* a physical object that can be experienced and approached as such (e.g., Slatman, 2008, pp. 81–82). Hence, phenomenological theories of health and illness that exclusively focus on the lived body are the mirror-image of naturalistic theories of health insofar as these reduce health to the subjective experience of the lived body. The crux for a more encompassing approach to health is the different aspects of the body, and search for how the interaction(s) between them constitute health and illness.

Phenomenological approaches to health and illness importantly counter approaches that primarily conceive of health and medicine in terms of institutionalised discourses. However, in doing so, they tend to conceive too much of the embodied experience of health as being isolated from a larger socio-cultural background. Because they tend to understand "the medical encounter" as being an encounter between doctor and patient, they threaten to lose out of sight that the ways in which individuals encounter "the medical" are way more complex than presupposed when taking the doctor-patient relationship as the central unit of medical practice. Furthermore, the prioritisation of lived experience as being primary to—or more authentic than—the practice of scientific objectification in medicine problematically presupposes a strict distinction between life in a biological (mechanistic) sense, and life as lived existentially.

Technological Embodiment

Now that I have sketched the general landscape of philosophical thought about health, it is important to return to what I indicated at the start of the introduction: the ideal of turning medicine into a preventive medicine and the role of technologies in the realisation of this shift. If the experience of healthy embodiment is indeed shaped by medical developments, the ideal of turning medicine into a preventive medicine should be taken into consideration. Since technological developments are thought to be key in realising this shift, analysing the constitution of healthy embodiment involves analysing how technologies are or can be incorporated into the embodied experience.

The technologies thought to be important for personalised medicine range from pacemakers to preventive screening to self-tracking technologies. Framed in terms of the approach taken in this book, such developments can be understood as shaping the experience of healthy embodiment. An important approach within the philosophy of technology that helps articulating the intertwinement of humans and technologies is postphenomenology. According to postphenomenologists, technologies should be understood as *mediating* the relationship that human beings have with the world around them (e.g., Ihde, 1990; Verbeek, 2005). Technologies are then understood as shaping how individuals experience and understand themselves and the world in which they are situated. They make present both the world and the individual relating to it in a specific way. For example, the use of obstetric ultrasound imaging in prenatal care mediates how unborn life becomes present to both physicians and expectant parents, thereby shaping what appear as relevant decisions concerning the unborn child (Verbeek, 2008).

The important issue to explore for this perspective is *how* specific technoscientific developments constitute both human beings and the world in which they live in a specific way—instead of being concerned with protecting human subjectivity against the objectifying and normalising tendencies of medical practice and/or technoscientific discourse. As a result, it does not make sense to think of "the body" as something existing outside of its relation with technoscientific developments. Rather than presupposing that entities such as "the body" or "the human being" do exist in isolation—and to which a primordiality or authenticity can be attributed, this perspective takes it as a starting point that such entities are the outcome of their relation with technologies and technoscientific discourses. Taking this perspective as a starting point implies that a philosophical exploration of health is always an exploration of how health is being shaped by technoscientific developments, such as the development of preventive medicine and the focus on lifestyle change it is accompanied with.

This exploration requires to make an analytic distinction between two aspects of technological mediation: on the one hand, it can be explored how they mediate relations between individuals and the environment—including other individuals. On the other hand, it can be explored how they mediate the relationship between individuals and their own bodies. As we will see in this book, this postphenomenological perspective proves relevant for understanding how medical technologies and the imaginaries around them shape the experience of healthy embodiment.

Healthy Embodiment: Towards a Systematic Account

The goal of this book is to provide an account of the embodied experience of health that does not reduce it to either a subjective experience, an objective description, or a form of normalisation. As I will attempt to show, the experience of health is constituted in the relationships between these different aspects of embodiment and the friction experienced within these relationships as well as in relation to the environment. This perspective enables connecting two strands of philosophical thinking about the body that are often kept apart: Foucauldian approaches on the one hand, and phenomenological approaches on the other. The former traditionally conceive of the body as the product of dominant social norms, whereas the latter consider the lived body as generating norms through habit formation (cf. Wehrle, 2017). By considering the lived (or experiential) body not as a separate entity but as an aspect of a body of which another aspect is constituted by social and biomedical norms, these two strands of thinking can be connected. Work in critical or feminist phenomenology has recently already started to connect these approaches to investigate how certain social expectations, technoscientific discourses, or other power structures shape (female) embodiment, as well as how these discourses and expectations can be used to silence and oppress marginalised groups (e.g., Guenther, 2021). However, to the best of my knowledge, whereas significant attention has been paid to how the combination of a Foucauldian and phenomenological approach to develop specific analyses of embodiment in particular (medical) contexts (e.g., de Boer & Zeiler, 2024; Zeiler & Folkmarson Käll, 2014), it has thus far not led to a general account of healthy embodiment, which is the main goal of this book.

The different chapters of the book navigate between these phenomenological and Foucauldian perspectives to identify different aspects of embodiment and the relationships between these aspects. This book is theoretical in nature and aims at giving a philosophical account of how the experience of healthy embodiment is constituted. The aim is to reveal how the body is constituted in its relation to medical norms such that a specific experience of health becomes possible. Roughly put, the starting point of my account is phenomenological, consistent with the focus on healthy embodiment. However, precisely because this book maintains that objectification is key to the experience of healthy embodiment, it moves on to the work of Foucault and addresses the extent to which medical practice exercises power over the bodies of individuals and how orienting to medical norms shapes the experience of health. How medical norms shape the experience of health is further illustrated by discussing the use of medical technologies and the project of personalised medicine.

Chapter 1 explores what kind of ontology of the body is put forward in the phenomenology of medicine and positions this ontology vis-à-vis the reductionist biomedical ontology of the body. I show how the concept of embodiment emerged out of the *Leib-Körper* distinction made by Husserl, was further expanded by Merleau-Ponty and Leder, and is taken up in contemporary phenomenology of medicine. I suggest that an important insight of Husserl has been lost in current phenomenology of medicine, namely that *Leib* and *Körper* are not mutually exclusive categories but that embodied experiences are constituted in the relationship between those different aspects of the body. Objectification, then, appears to be an intricate part of embodied experience. And, since we are not completely in charge of how we are objectified and experience our own body *as* objectified, an analysis of healthy embodiment cannot do without an analysis of how one's body is constituted in relation to the objectifying processes it is immersed in.

Chapter 2 introduces the idea that the 20th century marks the birth of a medicalised society. As a result of the objectification of the human body, all human activities have become potential objects of medical intervention. The work of Ivan Illich will be used to exemplify how one can conceive of this development as problematic by positing an idea(l) of health as being uncontaminated by medical activity. I suggest that one of the key problems in Illich's analysis is his premise that it is possible to make a distinction between medical and cultural-symbolic norms, such that the importance—or authenticity—of the latter can be stressed. On the basis of Foucault's work—particularly his critique of Illich—I argue that, precisely because we indeed live in a medicalised society, it is not possible to take recourse to extra-medical norms when understanding the experience of health. Instead, since medicalisation is grounded in a particular constitution of one's body as part of governable population, the embodied experience of being healthy inescapably ties in with an ontology of the body as part of a population.

Chapter 3 is concerned with the question of whether governmental control and the power that governments exercise in the end have the final say in distinguishing between health and illness, or between normal and abnormal. To answer this question, I engage with Foucault's analysis of power. In doing so, I show that power should not be understood as a force exercised from above that is to be understood as a form of domination, but instead as something productive. It creates a certain type of embodiment and subjectivity that is subjected to certain norms and values but is—precisely because it remains a form of subjectivity—itself productive too. This productivity resides in the potential to individually or collectively problematise the norms to which it is subject to; to engage in counter-conduct, as Foucault would call it. As a result, the experience of healthy embodiment cannot be reduced to the institutional or biomedical norms that partly constitute it, as the relationality of embodiment itself involves a productive principle.

Chapter 4 is concerned with how technologies are integrated into embodiment. I suggest that technologies are involved in the logic of governmentality and constitute power relations. Since the development of medicine relies on the use of medical technologies, ranging from pacemakers to self-tracking technologies, a key question is how such technologies shape the experience of healthy embodiment. In this chapter, I show that most accounts of technological embodiment maintain that technologies (1) allow for becoming transparent in embodied experience, (2) attain a high degree of transparency in virtue of this incorporation and (3) that the extent to which technological embodiment is considered to be healthy is understood to be relative to the degree of technological transparency. In contrast with such views, I suggest that technological transparency is neither possible nor desirable. Drawing from the work of Georges Canguilhem, I argue that the experience of health inevitably involves an experience of friction. This friction is experienced both due to the demands that (technological) environments put on the embodied subject, as well as due to the frictions emerging in the relationships between the different aspects of the body. Technologies, then, should not be understood in terms of their transparency but instead as introducing novel types of frictions that become part of the experience of healthy embodiment.

The final Chapter 5 specifically engages with the movement that can be loosely called *personalised medicine.* As I show in this chapter, personalised medicine is a loose umbrella-term referring to the ideal of making medical practice better tailored to the lives and bodies of individuals. As such, it can be considered to be a governmental practice. As the practical realisation of personalised medicine is far from complete or evident, I propose to understand it as what Jasanoff (2015) has called a *sociotechnical imaginary*: a perceived desirable future that is grounded in the perceived potentialities of technoscience that people can collectively work towards. This vision of an imagined future, then, has normative import in that it provides a blueprint of which behaviours are desirable in light of the possible realisation of the imagined future, thereby imposing certain institutional pressures on people to help bring this future about. Introducing the notion of sociotechnical imaginary serves to extend the main argument: the experience of healthy embodiment is not only shaped by a material healthcare infrastructure but also by the visions of what healthcare systems should look like and the role that individuals and (prospective) patients should play. This argument is strengthened through a critical discussion of the notion of empowerment that is often considered to be an important outcome of personalised medicine.

The concluding epilogue serves (1) to briefly situate the approach to healthy embodiment developed in this book in relation to neighbouring approaches, and (2) to identify the most important limits of this book and points to avenues for future research. I first position myself in relation to work that considers the (healthy) body as a network that lacks any core. Such accounts, often inspired by the work of Deleuze, deny that there is a more or less stable body that can function as a reference point and on which "health" can be predicated. Second, I address the question—for instance posed by Nikolas Rose—if Foucault's notion of the medical gaze is still sufficient to describe the influence of medical institutions in the 21st century, and stress the continuity between the medical gaze and what Rose terms the molecular gaze. Third, the epilogue explicates how the account of health developed in this book provides a starting point for analysing how the experience of health is intersubjectively shaped.

Note

1 At this point, it is my intention to discuss Boorse's naturalism on its own terms. Therefore, I will not develop an argument in favour of or against the idea that there can be such a thing as natural science without involving evaluative judgements. For an argument suggesting that natural science (the biomedical sciences included) inevitably involves evaluative and normative judgements, see: de Boer, te Molder, & Verbeek (2018).

References

Boenink, M. (2009). Tensions and opportunities in convergence: Shifting concepts of disease in emerging molecular medicine. *Nanoethics*, *3*(3), 243–255. https://doi.org/10.1007/s11569-009-0078-7

de Boer, B., te Molder, H., & Verbeek, P.P-. (2018). The perspective of the instruments: Mediating collectivity. *Foundations of Science*, *23*(4), 739–755. https://doi.org/10.1007/s10699-018-9545-3

de Boer, M., & Zeiler, K. (2024). Qualitative critical phenomenology. *Phenomenology and the Cognitive Sciences*. https://doi.org/10.1007/s11097-024-10034-7

Boorse, C. (1975). On the distinction between disease and illness. *Philosophy & Public Affairs*, *5*(1), 49–68.

Boorse, C. (1977). Health as a theoretical concept. *Philosophy of Science*, *44*(4), 542–573.

Boorse, C. (1997). A rebuttal on health. In J.M. Humber & R.F. Almeder (Eds.), *What is disease?* (pp. 3–134). Humana Press.

Canguilhem, G. (1991). *The normal and the pathological* (C.R. Fawcett, trans.). ZONE Books.

Carel, H. (2016). *Phenomenology of illness*. Oxford University Press.

Foucault, M. (1978). *The history of sexuality: Volume 1: An introduction* (R. Hurley, trans.). Pantheon Books.

Foucault, M. (1980). Body/Power. In C. Gordon (Ed.), *Power/Knowledge: Selected interviews and other writings 1972–1977* (pp. 55–62). Pantheon Books.

Gadamer, H.G-. (1996). *The enigma of health: The art of healing in a scientific age* (J. Gaiger & N. Walker, trans.). Polity Press.

Giroux, É. (2016). Introduction. Why a book on naturalism in the philosophy of health? In É. Giroux (Ed.), *Naturalism in the philosophy of health: Issues and implications* (pp. 1–16). Springer.

Guenther, L. (2021). Six sense of critique for critical phenomenology. *Puncta: Journal of Critical Phenomenology*, *4*(2), 5–23. https://doi.org/10.5399/pjcp.v4i2.2

Heidegger, M. (2001). *Zollikon seminars: Protocols-conversations-letters* (F. Mayr & R. Aslay, trans.). Northwestern University Press.
Ihde, D. (1990). *Technology and the lifeworld: From garden to earth*. Indiana University Press.
Jasanoff, S. (2015). Future imperfect. In S. Jasanoff & S.H-. Kim (Eds.), *Dreamscapes of modernity: Sociotechnical imaginaries and the fabrication of power* (pp. 1–33). The University of Chicago Press.
Kingma, E. (2014). Naturalism about health and disease: Adding nuance for progress. *Journal of Medicine and Philosophy*, *39*(6), 590–608. https://doi.org/10.1093/jmp/jhu037
Lupton, D. (2012). *Medicine as culture: Illness, disease and the body* (3rd ed.). SAGE
Metzl, J.M. (2010). Why "against health"?. In J.M. Metzl & A. Kirkland (Eds.), *Against health: How health became the new morality* (pp. 1–13). New York University Press.
Prainsack, B. (2017). *Personalized medicine: Empowered patients in the 21st century?* New York University Press.
Schramme, T. (2007). A qualified defence of a naturalistic theory of health. *Medicine, Health Care, and Philosophy*, *10*(1), 11–17. https://doi.org/10.1007/s11019-006-9020-8
Schütz, A. (2011). Reflections on the problem of relevance. In L. Embree (Ed.), *Alfred Schutz: Collected papers V. Phenomenology and the social sciences* (pp. 93–197). Springer.
Slatman, J. (2008). *Vreemd lichaam: Over medisch ingrijpen en persoonlijke identiteit*. AMBO.
Svenaeus, F. (2001). *The hermeneutics of medicine and the phenomenology of health: Steps towards a philosophy of medical practice*. Springer.
Vegter, M.W. (2018). Towards precision medicine: A new biomedical cosmology. *Medicine, Health Care, and Philosophy*, *21*(4), 443–456. https://doi.org/10.1007/s11019-018-9828-z
Verbeek, P.P-. (2005). *What things do: Philosophical reflections on technology, agency, and design* (R.P. Crease, trans.). The State University of Pennsylvania Press.
Verbeek, P.P-. (2008). Obstetric ultrasound and the technological mediation of morality: A postphenomenological analysis. *Human Studies*, *31*, 11–26. https://doi.org/10.1007/s10746-007-9079-0
Vogt, H., Hofmann, B., & Getz, L. (2016). The new holism: P4 systems medicine and the medicalization of health and life itself. *Medicine, Health Care, and Philosophy*, *19*(2), 307–323. https://doi.org/10.1007/s11019-016-9683-8
Wehrle, M. (2017). The normative body and the embodiment of norms: Bridging the gap between phenomenological and Foucauldian approaches. *Yearbook of Eastern and Western Philosophy*, *2*, 323–337. https://doi.org/10.1515/yewph-2017-0023
Welsh, T. (2022). *Feminist existentialism, biopolitics, and critical phenomenology in a time of bad health*. Routledge.
Zeiler, K., & Folkmarson Käll, K. (2014). *Feminist phenomenology and medicine*. State University of New York Press.

1 Our Two Bodies

Phenomenology, Health and Biomedicine

Introduction

The phenomenological method is typically presented in the form of a critique of medicine's naturalism and practices of objectification. For instance, according to Carel, medicine intends to develop naturalistic accounts of diseases (i.e., physiological dysfunction), thereby neglecting the experience of illness. Since the latter cannot be addressed through scientific objectification, medicine needs to be augmented with a focus on the lived experience of illness (Carel, 2016, p. 1). Similarly, Svenaeus holds that naturalism is accompanied with an image of health that equates it with the absence of diseases, thereby viewing it exclusively in biomedical terms. He argues that this image of health constitutes "a too narrow approach to the goal of clinical practice [...] [because while] to find diseases and to cure or mitigate them form significant *parts* of this activity, [...] the activity includes much more than that" (Svenaeus, 2001, p. 114). A phenomenology of health, then, should augment a naturalistic approach by articulating this "much more than that".

A central concern of phenomenological approaches is that medicine allegedly exhibits a biomedical gaze that functions as an *objectification apparatus* that eliminates a central aspect (i.e., subjective experiences) of health and illness from view. Since health is something that concerns the life of an individual as a whole, proponents of phenomenological accounts of health maintain that there is something essential to health that evades the ontology of the body that is put forward in the biomedical sciences. Since medical professionals are trained to exclusively view the human body in objective terms, so it is argued, lived experiences of health and illness are systematically treated as being irrelevant. Hence, an important goal of phenomenological analyses of health and illness is to carve out a space in medical practice in which the embodied experience of patients can be articulated.

In this chapter, I will critically evaluate to what extent phenomenology enables to provide a coherent account of health. Since health is considered

DOI: 10.4324/9781003602385-2

to be an embodied experience and taken to be (at least) partly the result of physiological processes inside the body, the key issue that guides my inquiry is what kind of ontology of the body is put forward in phenomenology. The critical question that can be derived from this issue is whether a phenomenological ontology of the body provides sufficient ground for the development of an account of health.

§1.1 The Body in the Phenomenological Tradition

Embodiment is an important topic in phenomenology. Analyses of embodiment often mobilise, in one way or another, the distinction between *Leib* and *Körper*. Roughly, the latter term refers to our body as an object in geometrical space that can be observed from a third-person perspective, that has certain measurable physiological characteristics and to which certain properties can be attributed. The former refers to our body as being lived and as making possible our experience of other entities and to project ourselves into the world. The differences that are expressed in the German words "Leib" and "Körper" are notoriously difficult to translate into English. For instance, in the translation of Husserl's *Ideas II*, Leib is translated as "Body", whereas Körper is translated as "body". More recent English translations try to capture the difference by using twin concepts such as "physical/material body" versus "lived/animated body", or "objective body" versus "subjective body" (Slatman, 2019). In either case, such conceptual pairs point to the different ways in which our body can be constituted for us, and what kind of different perspectives on it are possible. In the next three sections, I discuss three seminal analyses in the phenomenology of embodiment: those of Husserl, Merleau-Ponty and Leder. This discussion serves to develop an understanding of the different ways in which the body has been a topic of phenomenological inquiry and to enable the reader to judge which aspects of this inquiry are incorporated into the work of contemporary phenomenologists of medicine (introduced in §1.2).

§1.1.1 *Husserl and the Leib–Körper Distinction*

The question of the constitution of the body is important for Husserl because the body is itself a constitutive part of perception: "The Body [*Leib*] is, in the first place, the *medium of all perception*; it is the *organ of perception* and is *necessarily* involved in all perception [...and a] zero-point of orientation, the bearer of the here and the now, out of which the pure Ego intuits space and the whole world of the senses" (Husserl, 1989, p. 61). Husserl's more specific analysis of the body serves to investigate the "constitution of this Corporeality" that correlates with every experience (Husserl, 1989, p. 152). It is in this context that Husserl distinguishes between two different ways of *apprehending* corporeality, by pointing to the different ways in which it can be constituted for a consciousness.

The starting point for Husserl's analysis is the famous example of touching one's own left hand. When I touch my left hand with my right hand, I perceive some qualities of my left hand (e.g., a certain shape, a certain smoothness, a certain warmth), but at the same time, my left hand also *senses* that it is being touched: the act of touching produces certain sensations in my left hand that are localised on the very hand being touched. On the basis of this example, Husserl develops the seminal distinction between *Leib* and *Körper*: "[T]he Body is originally constituted in a double way: first, it is a physical thing, *matter*; it has its extension, in which are included its real properties, its colour, smoothness, hardness, warmth, and whatever other material qualities of that kind there are. Second, I find on it, and I *sense* "on" it and "in" it: warmth on the back of the hand, coldness in the feet, sensations of touch in the fingertips" (Husserl, 1989, p. 153). One's body, accordingly, can never be constituted by mere matter because it senses certain appearances that have their own *localisation* on it. That is, when touching corporeality, this touch has a particularly localised "place" on it, which gives rise to certain sensations.

Shortly after establishing that, in terms of localisation, two different ways of apprehending corporeality can be distinguished, Husserl notes that the same way of distinguishing cannot be established when corporeality is approached with the visual senses: "Obviously, the Body is also to be seen just like any other thing, but it becomes a *Body* only by incorporating tactile sensations, pain sensations, etc.—in short, by the localisation of the sensations as sensations" (Husserl, 1989, pp. 158–159). When perceiving my body through my visual senses, I am unable to localise sensations as sensations, such that a double apprehension does not take place. In the act of seeing, I do not apprehend my eyes as something seeing that is simultaneously seen. In this sense, it is only in tactility that corporeality can be constituted as being both *Leib* and *Körper*, such that it becomes clear these different ways of apprehension are fundamentally intertwined and form a union that can be called a *LeibKörper* (e.g., Husserl, 1989, p. 170).

The fact that one's body has the unique feature of being a field of localisation makes it that not only its own constitution can be understood in terms of the distinction between *Leib* and *Körper*, but that it ultimately grounds any perception of other material things. That is, these things can only be observed to the extent that they enter the field of localisation presupposed in embodiment. As Husserl puts it: "The subject, constituted as counter-member of material nature, is [...] an Ego, to which a Body belongs as a field of localization of its sensations. The Ego has the 'faculty' (the 'I can') to freely move this Body—i.e., the organ in which it is articulated—and to perceive an external world by means of it" (Husserl, 1989, pp. 159–160). The additional step that Husserl takes here is that the body is not a stationary object, but instead perceives the external world through the ability of movement that constitutes the possibility that other entities enter one's body's field of localisation.

The non-stationary nature of one's own body is grounded in what Husserl calls the "I can". A fundamental feature of embodiment is that the body moves through the world as a field of localisation on which different sensations can be localised. Perception is not grounded in an absolute stationary consciousness for which representations happen to pass by, but instead in the lived experience of sensations that are localised on the body. As a result, in an act of perception, "movements of the body and of the eyes do not enter into the picture as real processes of nature, but instead a domain of possibilities of free movement is most properly present to me" (Husserl, 1989, p. 228). Our relation with other objects, then, is constituted by the faculty of the "I can". Crucially, the "I can" is not a property that consciousness projects onto the body, but instead is the only manner in which it is possible to grasp any relationship with intentional objects: "In the 'I can' there obviously resides not merely a representation but, beyond that, a thesis, one which thereby concerns not only myself but also the 'doing', not the actual doing but precisely the being able to do so" (Husserl, 1989, p. 273).

By following Husserl's analysis of embodiment that leads to the distinction between *Leib* and *Körper*, we have discovered two ways in which embodiment enables the constitution of our relation to other objects. First, it is through tactility that it becomes clear that *Leib* and *Körper* form a union, as well as that those are two different modes of apprehending corporeality. This is why any relationship with an object presupposes that it enters the body's field of localisation and that there are different ways in which objects can do so. Second, since embodiment presupposes the possibility of movement that is conceptualised in terms of the "I can", the field of localisation is not stable but instead results from the body's possibility of movement that enables it to encounter objects that are localised. In conjunction, these show how we must understand Husserl's claim that the body is a medium for all perception in *Ideas II*.

§1.1.2 Merleau-Ponty: The Worldly Character of Embodiment

The *Leib–Körper* distinction gained further prominence—although in slightly different terms—by how it was incorporated into Merleau-Ponty's work, who makes embodiment the cornerstone of his phenomenology. Merleau-Ponty takes Husserl's analysis of the body in a somewhat different direction. For Husserl, the (often incomplete) constitution of corporeality points to a problem of how certain aspects of the world appear to consciousness. According to Husserl, the body, "which serves me as means for all my perception obstructs me in the perception of itself and is a remarkably imperfectly constituted thing" (Husserl, 1989, p. 167). Merleau-Ponty, however, understands humans not as *having* bodies that have peculiar phenomenological features, but instead as *being* bodies that can only project themselves into the world in virtue of embodiment.

The point here is not to argue in favour or against a strong divide between the phenomenological approaches of Husserl and Merleau-Ponty. Rather, it is my purpose to show that, in the work of Merleau-Ponty, a transition can be detected by which the question of the body's constitution is replaced by the question of how the world is constituted in virtue of embodiment.[1] Put differently, for Merleau-Ponty, it is not so much the constitution of *LeibKörper* through localisation that is of phenomenological relevance, but rather Husserl's insight that embodiment always presupposes an "I can".

In *The Phenomenology of Perception*, Merleau-Ponty places great emphasis on how perception is grounded in the embodiment, which "is the vehicle of being-in-the-world [through which we are] united with a definite milieu, merg[e] with certain projects, and [are] perpetually engaged therein" (Merleau-Ponty, 2012, p. 84). This experience of embodiment is, in line with Husserl, contrasted with body's appearance as a three-dimensional object in geometrical space when approached from a third-person perspective. As Merleau-Ponty puts it: "I am not the result or the intertwining of multiple causalities that determine my body or my 'psyche'; I cannot think of myself as a part of the world, like the simple object of biology, psychology and sociology; I cannot enclose myself within the universe of science" (Merleau-Ponty, 2012, pp. lxxi–lxxii).

Whereas Merleau-Ponty, again in alignment with Husserl, does not deny that it is possible to observe human bodies from a third-person perspective, he takes this perspective to be incapable of getting what is most essential about the human body into view. First and foremost, so Merleau-Ponty maintains, the body must be understood in terms of an "I can" (Merleau-Ponty, 2012, p. 139), thereby disclosing the world in such a way that I can smoothly carry out the movements needed to pursue my goals and projects. Our body is a vehicle for action through which the world in which we live becomes meaningful. This emphasis marks a slight difference with Husserl, who initially asked how the body is constituted for consciousness and remarks that we can only understand the constitution of the body as *LeibKörper* with reference to tactuality. Merleau-Ponty, in contrast, suggests that when analysing the body's constitution, "I am not in front of my body, I am in my body, or rather I am my body. [...] I do not simply contemplate the relations between the segments of my body and the correlation between my visual body and my tactile body; rather, I am myself the one who holds these arms and legs together, the one who simultaneously sees them and touches them" (Merleau-Ponty, 2012, p. 151). The "I can" is not so much a faculty of the Ego as it is for Husserl, but rather points to the inseparability of body and world: the body is always already the body that I inhabit and through which the world appears to me as meaningful in the first place.

If embodiment is primarily understood in terms of the "I can", how can we analyse its constitution? According to Merleau-Ponty, the notions of motor intentionality and habit are crucial in this respect.[2] Because Merleau-Ponty characterises embodiment in terms of an "I can", he singles out motricity as the primary mode of intentionality (Merleau-Ponty, 2012, p. 139). Inhabiting a world implies a familiarity with the objects around us and the capacity to interact with them without any prior representation. Concretely, when reaching for an object (say, a glass), we are not imagining beforehand what is the exact distance between my body and the object, but rather respond immediately to the object's solicitation without any mediating representations. Motricity, then, "is not [...] a servant of consciousness, transporting the body to the point of space that we imagine beforehand" (Merleau-Ponty, 2012, p. 140). Rather, we position ourselves in the environment through what Merleau-Ponty calls a *body schema*: a pre-reflective unconscious manner of experiencing the environment and one's capacities to act in it (see also: Gallagher 1986). This fundamental characteristic, then, is also why one's body resists being completely captured in an objectifying third-person scientific point of view and is never completely constituted for the experiencing subject: "What prevents it [my body] from ever being an object or from ever being 'completely constituted' is that my body is that by which there are objects" (Merleau-Ponty, 2012, p. 94).

In embodied experience, our body can hence not be described as a collection of different organs and limbs in geometrical space, but should instead be considered a whole in which the different senses (e.g., touching, hearing, seeing) are integrated (e.g., Ihde, 2002, p. 38). This body schema forms the horizon for how other objects appear to me and shapes the possibilities for perception and action (i.e., the "I can"). The body schema is not something static, not something that remains the same over a lifetime, but is instead dynamic in that is modified in light of past experiences and actions, as well as the objective properties of the body (e.g., the body schema might change when someone loses a leg). It is always constituted in relation to the specific situatedness of the embodied individual and is acquainted through habit and sedimentation: "my own body is the primordial *habit*, the one that conditions all others and by which they can be understood" (Merleau-Ponty, 2012, p. 93, my emphasis).

When moving through my hometown to do some grocery shopping, I know the directions to the grocery store around the corner without having to make them explicit. I do not need to contemplate where the store is exactly located and which other objects (e.g., houses, garbage cans) I need to pass to arrive there. When going down the stairs, I do not need to recall the distance between the respective steps, nor do I need to explicitly establish the distance that I am about to travel when leaving the door of the house. The world that I inhabit as an embodied subject already presupposes the presence of a relationship between a manifold of virtual coordinates that do not need to be made explicit (Merleau-Ponty, 2012, p. 131). These virtual coordinates are not properties of an external world waiting to be found by the embodied individual, but are the result of a process of *sedimentation* through which the world is constituted in the first place.

Merleau-Ponty stresses that the notion of sedimentation should not lead us back to a covert representationalism through which my trip to the grocery store is understood as the result of a series of strongly connected mental images. Instead, the possibility for my unproblematic trip to the grocery store "only remains around me as my familiar domain if I still hold 'in my hands' or 'in my legs' its principal distances and directions, and only if a multitude of intentional threads run out towards it from my body" (Merleau-Ponty, 2012, pp. 131–132). Put differently, sedimentation is grounded in motricity but in turn shapes how motor intentionality concretely manifests such that a familiar world is constituted.

The entanglement of sedimentation and motor intentionality simultaneously implies that the ability to enter a meaningful world depends both on the physical constitution of one's body and on the body's lived history. This interplay becomes dramatically visible in novels such as Franz Kafka's *The Metamorphosis* or Philip Roth's *The Breast*, or in the many examples of pathologies discussed in the *Phenomenology of Perception*. The tragedy of Gregor Samsa in *The Metamorphosis* not only consists in his transformation into a huge insect, but first and foremost in his inability—and the inability of the people close to him—to maintain (or regain) a meaningful world after Gregor's transformation. Gregor's interactions with the objects and others around him have lost their initial meaning, which makes him unable to continue anticipating on the projects that he used to anticipate on. And the other way around, his appearance prevents—as exemplified in his interactions with his sister Grete—others from integrating him into their lives against a familiar horizon. Gregor's being-in-the-world and intentional relationship with the entities around him loses its meaning because of his bodily modification that initiates an abrupt break with his initial pattern of sedimentation. In the absence of a novel pattern of sedimentation that synchronises with his novel bodily appearance, Gregor ends up in a situation in which all his previous have lost their meaning and can no longer be interpreted against a novel horizon of familiarity.

Towards the end of the novel, Gregor dies of starvation—which separates him from any form of being-in-the-world—and his struggle ends.

From a phenomenological point of view, the tragedy of Kafka's story can be interpreted in terms of a sudden loss of a familiar form of embodiment that can be explained by a mismatch between Gregor's physical bodily capacities and his previous pattern(s) of sedimentation. And the tragedy remains to be present throughout the novel because Gregor continuously experiences that he is stuck in a particular form of embodiment that breaks with any previous horizon, while simultaneously remaining to interpret the situations which he is in against this previous horizon. In this relationship between motor intentionality and sedimentation, it becomes clear that any perception and experience are grounded in embodiment and that embodiment can never be transcended completely in that any meaningful horizon is a correlate of one's bodily possibilities.

Merleau-Ponty expresses the idea that one's body is the condition of possibility of intentionality, but that intentionality simultaneously lacks any essential characteristics as follows: "My body is this meaningful core that behaves as a general function and that nevertheless exists and that is susceptible to illness" (Merleau-Ponty, 2012, p. 48). One's body usually is the vehicle by means of which one is able to live in a meaningful place without noticing it explicitly, because it is the function as a result of which one's world is constituted. At the same time, however, the body is vulnerable to illness such that it can become the centre of our focus and the vehicle through which the things around us appear as *unfamiliar*. In either case, the body remains constitutive of how we experience the world: "What allows us to center our existence is also what prevents us from centering it completely, and the anonymity of our body is inseparably both freedom and servitude" (Merleau-Ponty, 2012, p. 87). Hence, one's body is both the vehicle for developing habits and patterns of sedimentation and the very thing through which existing habits and orientations are disrupted.

Further developing the Husserlian discovery of embodiment in *Ideas II*, Merleau-Ponty takes the "I can"—the possibility of movement and anticipation—to be the core of any intentional relationship with the world. Embodiment is for Merleau-Ponty not something that can be made an object for an Ego, but is the condition of possibility for any form of being-in-the-world. This analysis of embodiment in terms of motor intentionality and sedimentation can be considered as an extension of Husserl's analysis of the body as a site of localisation in the sense that Merleau-Ponty investigates *how* the body is constituted *as* a field of localisation. As a result, he does not depart—as Husserl seems to do—from the idea that something as a stationary body is conceivable and of which it subsequently can be concluded that it presupposes movement, but instead takes as a starting point that to exist presupposes to inhabit a world. The existence of this world is dependent on the body in that it is constituted in the relationship between motor intentionality and sedimentation. Hence, for Merleau-Ponty, any analysis of embodiment is not so much an analysis of the body itself, but instead of one's relation to the environment and the patterns of sedimentation that structure this relation.

§*1.1.3 Leder: The Absent Body*

Our last stop in discussing 20th century analyses of embodiment is Drew Leder's 1990 book *The Absent Body*. His work is of relevance to our discussion because it shows how the 20th century "discovery" of the body in phenomenological philosophy essentially implies a discovery of the body's *absence*: "While in one sense the body is the most abiding and inescapable presence in our lives, it is also essentially characterized by absence" (Leder, 1990b, p. 1). While thus largely siding with Husserl's and Merleau-Ponty's analyses that one's body is absent—in that it remains unthematised—when carrying out our projects, Leder intends to qualify the different ways in which bodies can be absent. For Leder, this project is important for the phenomenology of embodiment for at least two reasons: (1) insofar as the phenomenological project can be considered as an attempt to overcome Cartesian dualism, overemphasising or ontologising the distinction between *Leib* and *Körper* re-affirms dualistic thought and hence runs counter to the very aims of phenomenology (Leder, 1990b, p. 6), and (2) qualifying different modes of absence enables to articulate how the body's physiology and objectivity shape one's being-in-the-world.

Leder's criticisms—or augmentations—of Husserl and Merleau-Ponty are good entry points to his work. As we saw earlier, Husserl describes the body as the medium for all perception and as a zero-point [*Nullpunkt*] for orientation. For Leder, this latter metaphor is misleading for two reasons: one's body "is never a pure nullity in experience, but neither is it simply a point" (Leder, 1990b, pp. 23–24). What would it mean for one's body to be a pure nullity? This would imply, Leder maintains, that the body is fully eradicated from the experiential world. However, I always experience myself as situated in the here and now, as within a certain vicinity or distance of surrounding objects that have different degrees of accessibility (Leder, 1990b, p. 23). When I want to open a door at the other end of the room, I am well aware that I have to take a couple of steps before I can reach it and already anticipate interacting with the doorknob. This implies that I do explicitly not experience myself as a total nullity, but instead as situated amongst the things around me.

Yet, the fact that I always experience myself as situated here should not lure us into understanding one's body as a point on a geometrical plane. For Leder, this is immediately clear from the fact that it is perfectly possible to attain a *perspective on aspects of one's body*; for instance, I can move my hand in front of my face or touch my eyes with my hands and sense my body differently when taking such different perspectives: this would not be possible if the body would just be a point in geometrical space. These different perspectives can never be combined into the perception of an integrated whole or a complete thematisation of the body, but, and this is how Leder critically relates to Husserl: the fact that the body can never be *fully* thematised does not necessarily imply that it cannot be thematised *at all*. A phenomenological exploration of the body should therefore focus on the different ways in which one's body can be absent and present.

Leder's critique of Merleau-Ponty focuses on how embodiment cannot be exhaustively explained in terms of the "I can". As we saw in the previous section, Merleau-Ponty describes the "I can" in terms of motor intentionality and sedimentation that are constitutive of world. Leder agrees with Merleau-Ponty in that the absence of an explicit experience *of* our body is a condition of possibility for inhabiting the world and engaging in (meaningful) action. My actions and habits, then, "are enveloped within the structure of the taken-for-granted body from which I *inhabit* the world" (Leder, 1990b, p. 32). The ordinary way of inhabiting a world, then, is one in which my body allows me to engage in actions without becoming an object of attention itself, a phenomenon Leder captures with the notion of the "absent presence" of the body (Leder, 1990b, p. 13).

Leder links this absent presence to the bodily structure of the "I can" that Merleau-Ponty puts forward as the body's fundamental capacity in the *Phenomenology of Perception*: ordinary being-in-the-world presupposes the presence of a bodily structure that is characterised by an absence. Augmenting Merleau-Ponty, Leder makes a distinction between two levels of bodily absence: the *surface level* and the *depth level*. The "I can" refers to the surface level of the body that is experientially unavailable because it is constitutive of any perceptual or sensory field (e.g., I cannot see my eyes that are constitutive of the screen that I am looking at, or I do not experience my legs explicitly when playing soccer). In Leder's analysis of embodiment, the "I can" is only one way in which embodiment manifests, namely in terms of *ekstasis*.

There is another aspect of the body, Leder maintains, that is equally constitutive of our experience and that is to be found in the "depth" of my body (Leder, 1990b, p. 36). The visceral aspects of my body, the functioning of my organs, or the physiological processes taking place in my body do texture how I experience the world and do so in virtue of their absence. However, this absence is different from the absence of the body surface: "The liver experientially disappears precisely because it is not the origin of any sensory field. It does not disappear in the act of perceiving, as does the eye, but by virtue of its withdrawal from the perceptual circuit" (Leder, 1990a, p. 217). On the basis of this distinction, Leder argues that we must distinguish between an "I can" characterised by the absence of the surface body and an "it can" that must be understood as the present absence of the body on a visceral level (Leder, 1990a, p. 212, 1990b, pp. 46–47). Both of these are crucial for my capacity to transcend into a meaningful world.

Whereas I have a relative degree of control over my surface body—this is characteristic of the "I can", the depths of my body are beyond my control, invisible to me, and work in ways that I have not voluntarily chosen.[3] Leder calls this aspect of the body the *recessive body*: "the body not only projects outwards in experience, but also falls back into unexperienceable depths" (1990b, p. 53). Framed in terms of the distinction between *Leib* and *Körper*, the recessive aspects can be understood as the body's inevitable objectivity (*Körper*) that nevertheless is constitutive of embodied experience (*Leib*). Even more, the present absence of the visceral body is—on Leder's account—a precondition for the "I can" experienced in healthy life: "The hiddenness of vital organs, though frustrating at times of disease, is essential to healthy functioning" (Leder, 1990b, p. 44).

This last observation brings Leder to the final form of qualified absence in embodiment: the *dys-appearing body*. This mode of absence reveals itself when I am in pain or suffer from disease. In such cases, "[t]he body is no longer a nullpoint but an active presence whose call we must resist" (Leder, 1990b, p. 76). For instance, when I am taking a walk through the woods and my back suddenly starts to hurt, my initial field of experience (that might consist of my conversational partner, the presence of nice trees or mushrooms, etc.) is turned over and replaced by a complete focus on my back, which now becomes the central core of my new field of experience. Suddenly, I am no longer able to enjoy my surroundings and/or to engage in a meaningful conversation, as I am immersed in the experience of pain and the accompanied desire for the pain to be removed. Depending on the duration and intensity of the pain, I might wait for it to leave or might actively look for help. In either case, the pain constitutes a new field of experience either through the explicit thematisation of the part of my body that is in pain or by the constitution of a new set of actions revolving around my pain's disappearance.

While in the case of pain it is possible that the feeling of pain disappears suddenly and that a "normal" field of experience appears again, the experience of disease is characterised by a longer period of experienced dysfunction as well as an uncertainty about the prospect of recovery. As I will discuss this experience more extensively in the next section, I move immediately to how Leder conceptualises the body's absence in cases of pain and disease. For Leder, the bodily mode of *dys-appearance* signifies the appearance of the body as demanding thematisation in virtue of its non-functioning. The body, then, does not so much *disappear* from view, but instead *appears* in a "dys-" state, in a state in which the occasional present absence of the body is pierced through (Leder, 1990b, p. 84). Thinking back to the example of Gregor Samsa in the previous section, this state can be understood as a radical break with previous patterns of sedimentation that are replaced by a novel field of experience, which can be, using Leder's vocabulary, fruitfully described in terms of bodily dys-appearance.

On the basis of this discussion of Leder's different modes of bodily absence, we can reconstruct a pattern in phenomenological analyses of embodiment in the 20th century. In Husserl, we find a discovery of the body as a zero-point of orientation that is presupposed in how the empirical Ego experiences its surroundings and of which the constitution can be phenomenologically analysed. On the basis of this analysis, Husserl distinguishes between two aspects of the body—*Leib* and *Körper*—that form a necessary synthesis: the *LeibKörper*. Merleau-Ponty radicalises Husserl's methodology in that he takes the empirical Ego as a starting point and rules out the possibility of any form of transcendental phenomenological analysis. As a result, he interprets the body in terms of an embodied "I can" that can only be analysed in terms of its interactions with its surroundings.

Leder, in turn, intends to return to the body's physicality that loses its importance in Merleau-Ponty's analysis. He intends to make bodily absence explicit by pointing to the layers of depth and invisibility that are presupposed in embodied intentionality. Besides the "I can", which is characteristic of the *ecstatic body*, Leder distinguishes the *recessive body* that is characterised by the body's visceral depth and the *dys-appearing body* that is characterised by the bodily appearance of non-functioning. Both of these aspects point to bodily powers that contribute to our embodied experience but that we have not chosen for and that we cannot completely control or fathom. This trajectory indicates that the phenomenological discovery of the body's presence leads up to a discovery of the body's absence that only comes explicitly to the fore in instances of dys-appearance.

In contemporary Western societies, the experience of bodily dys-appearance is typically connected with hospital visits, treatment plans and interactions with medical professionals. Leder describes the purpose of these interactions in terms of a search for the causes of pain and disease through a hermeneutic investigation of the depths of the visceral body. This investigation involves conversations between patients and medical professionals and the use of all kinds of imaging technologies to observe the body's visceral depths. The phenomenology of medicine and health, as we will see in the next section, typically takes as a starting point that such interactions often involve an objectification of the human body that must be critiqued.

§1.2 The Biomedical Gaze: A Phenomenological Critique

The starting point of phenomenological analyses of health and illness is the idea that there is a fundamental distinction between the objectifying third-person perspective on the human body prevalent in medicine, and the lived experience of the body from a first-person perspective. The need for criticising the objectifying third-person perspective is often justified with reference to the distinction between *Leib* and *Körper:* since the body's ontology cannot be exclusively captured in terms of its object-character (*Körper*), any attempt to interpret the body in objective terms inevitably fails to develop a complete view onto the body. And insofar as this objectifying view on the body is leading in medicine and removes the experience of being a body (*Leib*) from view, it should be corrected by a method that does justice to the body's ontological status. Phenomenology, then, is presented as the method that is capable of doing this job.

The relevance of phenomenology for medicine is thus justified by the claims (1) that biomedicine tends to objectify the human body, (2) that this form of objectification is grounded in a flawed ontology, and (3) that phenomenology enables one to articulate those aspects of embodiment relevant to health and illness that the medical sciences miss out on. In the next two sections, I will briefly discuss the work of two prominent phenomenologists of medicine: Havi Carel and Fredrik Svenaeus. These discussions serve as a starting point for critically evaluating how the phenomenology of medicine justifies its relevance.

§1.2.1 Health, Illness and Bodily Certainty

According to Carel, the experience of the healthy body is characterised by its *transparency*. For example, when eating, what I experience are neither the bodily movements required to move food from my plate into my mouth, nor do I explicitly thematise how my digestive system processes what I am eating. Instead, I am engaged in the activity of eating and immersed in the taste of the food without paying attention to the bodily movements and processes involved in this activity. Accordingly, although my body always is both subject and object, I do not experience it *as* an object in the ordinary flow of life.

Carel draws an analogy between the transparency of our body in health and Heidegger's phenomenology of tool use. Heidegger makes a distinction between present-at-hand entities and ready-to-hand entities. According to him, we do not relate to the tools we use as object in front of us (i.e., as present-at-hand), but we rather experience the world *through* them when pursuing our projects. It is only when tools cease to work that they appear as present-at-hand entities that are explicitly thematised as objects (e.g., Heidegger, 1985, §§15–16). For example, when I am writing a letter,

I do not experience the pen I use to write, but experience the surface of the piece of paper that I am writing on through the pen, while being immersed in the activity of writing a letter. It is only when the pen stops working properly that it is explicitly thematised as an object of attention, inviting questions such as: "why does this object prevent me from further engagement in my project?".

Carel extends Heidegger's analysis of the breakdown of tools to the body when inviting to "imagine that the pen works perfectly but I cannot use my hand [...]". She argues that "in these cases, too, I experience a failure of a tool, but this time the tool is part of my body" (Carel, 2016, p. 61). Carel's point is of course not to place bodily disfunctioning and the breakdown of a tool on equal footing, but rather to build on Heidegger's phenomenology of tool use to show how bodily disfunctioning modifies our experience of the world. The crucial difference that becomes visible when Heidegger's phenomenology of tool use is extended to the human body is that disfunctioning body parts (often) remain attached to the human body and tend to become increasingly disabling. Because of this, bodily disfunctioning has a profoundly different temporal dimension than the breakdown of a tool and has the potential to transform our experience and understanding of ourselves and the environment definitively. What this points to is that our experience of the world in health is dependent on the integrity of our bodies, such that disruptions of this integrity reveals the contingency of our everyday relation with the world (Carel, 2016, p. 62). Only when our body becomes a burden do we thematise our body as an object that influences our relationship with the environment.

Carel argues that simple bodily disruptions such as a cold or headache do not radically transform our healthy, everyday being in the world, because these still appear within a totality of *bodily certainty*. That is, "we feel tacitly confident (or rather, we do not normally question) that our bodies will continue to function in a similar fashion in which they have in the past" (Carel, 2016, p. 89). The habits that we have developed throughout our lives constitute a meaningful whole that is not directly experienced, yet implicitly offer a horizon against which the things we experience and the projects we engage in appear. For example, I expect that my legs will be able to walk me to the bus station this afternoon, which allows me to travel back home and play football in the evening. While I usually do not reflect on this, it is constitutive of how I understand my relation to myself and the environment. Also, when I am suffering from a headache, these activities remain to appear within a similar meaningful whole. It might take slightly longer to walk to the bus stop or be somewhat less pleasant, or even I must skip football practice today. Yet, I remain to expect that next week or the week after I can perform these activities again. Also in such cases, the world remains familiar to me because I tacitly assume that

I am capable of remaining to execute such habits and expect that my body does not disrupt the routinely habitual way through which I understand myself and my environment.

Carel thus conceives of health as a state of harmony between objective and subjective body, such that the former is transparent due to a sense of bodily certainty. This harmony makes possible the effortless execution of developed habits and constitutes a bodily certainty that makes it that we take it for granted that we can remain doing so in the future. As such, our body *as* a healthy body refrains from becoming an object of experience. Instead, *through* it, we experience and understand ourselves and the world in an unproblematic manner, thereby orienting to a meaningful horizon that allows for the planning and carrying out of our projects.

§*1.2.2 Health as Homelikeness*

In this section, I will turn to the work of Fredrik Svenaeus in order to analyse if a phenomenology of health can depart "from within health". Svenaeus draws on the work of Martin Heidegger to show that our everyday engagement with the world already offers a foundation for a phenomenology of health. Just as Carel characterises health in terms of the transparency of the body, Svenaeus maintains that health is something we transparently live *through*, instead of something that we consciously attend to. Therefore, a phenomenology of health requires an investigation of "the meaning of human experience situated in the world as acting, attuned, and embodied" (Svenaeus, 2001, p. 82). He takes Heidegger's work as a starting point and maintains that human beings (*Dasein*) are best understood in terms of their being-in-the-world. First and foremost, the world does not appear to a human being as an external object, but as an already meaningful totality to which (s)he is open to. As a result of this openness, the totality appears as a pattern for acting, thinking, feeling and talking. Crucial for Svenaeus—and Heidegger—is that understanding a totality as meaningful is not a cognitive disposition that can be explicitly articulated, but a form of *attunement*. To understand, then, "is to find one's place in the meaning-structure of the world and project oneself towards possible goals" (Svenaeus, 2001, p. 88).

However, at the same time, individuals are never fully familiar with (i.e., at home in) their world because it is shared with other individuals and a nature that somehow resists understanding. Our familiarity with the world is always "pervaded by a homelessness" (Svenaeus, 2001, p. 93) that threatens to alienate us from our everyday being-at-the-world. Being healthy, according to Svenaeus, consists in the ability to keep this alienation at bay; it "is to be understood as a being at home that keeps the not being at home in the world from becoming apparent" (Svenaeus, 2001, p. 93). Accordingly, health is not an entity that can be pointed at, or a specific state of affairs that can be analysed, but is a *process* of homelike attunement in which being-at-home is balanced with not-being-at-home such that our experience of being-in-the-world is one of familiarity and continuity.

Because health is defined as a balancing process, Svenaeus claims that health can be phenomenologically accessed by analysing the balance between homelikeness and unhomelikeness. Following Zaner (1981), the body is understood as being uncanny (*unheimlich*) in that it can always appear as strange to me, while clearly remaining part of my own context of experience. This strangeness can manifest in illness, when the body appears as something uncontrollable, but also in experiences like hunger or thirst, or by the way others might relate to it. In all such cases, the body remains familiar to me but at the same time displays a strangeness in that I still experience it in terms of a sense of otherness (Burwood, 2008). The experience of health, then, results in the balancing act of familiarity and otherness.

He compares the experience of health with riding a bicycle during which your balance may be challenged due to the surface you are riding on, and in reaction to which you will attempt to regain balance in order not to fall down, successfully or not (Svenaeus, 2001, p. 95). Similarly, our balancing can be challenged when experiencing an episode of migraine, during which the world is no longer familiar because vision is blurred and light no longer appears as a transparent source allowing us to engage in our daily activities (e.g., walking, typing), but instead as a source of frustration that increases the intensity of the migraine episode. In such moments, we are attuned with the world in such a way that it no longer appears as familiar (i.e., as homelike). What was previously experienced as background now actively penetrates into our world, making our world appear as something to which we do not belong to. The balance between homelikeness and unhomelikeness is in such an episode of migraine temporarily distorted, such that our "not being at home in the world" becomes apparent, only to disappear from understanding when the migraine episode is no longer experienced.[4] In other words, the experience of not being able to transcend *into* a meaningful world reveals the presence of a form of ordinary homelike attunement characterised by "the normal unapparent transparency of everyday activities" (Svenaeus, 2013, p. 234).

Whether experiences of illness—such as migraine episodes—can be considered experiences of unhomelikeness depends on the extent to which they prevent returning to a mood of homelike attunement. When an episode of migraine has passed by, one often manages to return to an understanding of the world within which previous projects can be continued, and no major disruptions of experience has taken place. That is, one returns to the harmonious rhythm of healthy being-in-the-world (Svenaeus, 2001, p. 99).

In contrast, experiences of illness—and this is what distinguishes them from episodes of temporary unhomelike attunement—disrupt the constitution of homelike attunement more permanently.

Phenomenological access to health is, on Svenaeus's account, thus grounded in the ability to sense that one is no longer at home in the world that one is attuned to, such that one is prevented from transcending to a meaningful world (2019, p. 464). As a result, the lack of self-evidence of the rhythm of one's life can become an object of reflection, precisely because it is no longer a self-evident background attunement that one transparently lives through.

§1.2.3 Subjectivity and Objectivity in the Phenomenology of Medicine

Recall the three ways in which the phenomenology of medicine justifies it relevance: (1) biomedicine tends to objectify the human body, (2) this form of objectification is grounded in a flawed ontology and (3) phenomenology enables to articulate those aspects of embodiment relevant to health and illness that the medical sciences miss out on. Let us now critically evaluate these claims in light of the above discussion.

Does biomedicine indeed tend to objectify the human body? Consider the following example that describes a woman giving birth in a hospital:

> "That really, really hurts", says the woman who has just given birth. The doctor is sitting by her splayed feet, which rest on stirrups either side of him. [...] She repeats: "That hurts. Are you using anaesthetic?". "No", the doctor replies calmly, "there is no need to. I'm nearly finished". The woman is too exhausted to persist and she says nothing more. It is hard to imagine another situation in which we would not offer pain relief to someone having a needle pushed through their genitals. But in this case the woman's testimony is not acted upon. Her pain is either not fully registered or not considered worthy of response.
>
> (Carel & Kidd, 2014, p. 529)

Clearly, this example from medical practice indicates how the human body can be objectified in medical practice in the sense that certain experiences (e.g., the woman's pain) are ignored by medical practitioners. The woman's body is (implicitly) perceived as a manipulable object whose experience are secondary to the goal being pursued. Although the above example is particularly cruel, there are many other ways in which human beings can be objectified in medical practice (Svenaeus, 2023). For instance, doing an x-ray scan or even being examined by a stethoscope are premised on the idea that the body's objectivity is relevant for addressing the complaints of patients, and assume that the verbal subjective reports of people do not tell the complete story about their bodies. In principle, there seems to be nothing wrong with objectification being a part of medical practice, as it can be in line with the patient's desire to find out what are the cause(s) of their medical problems and to develop a treatment plan that enables to address them.

I hope that the above examples are sufficiently convincing for us to accept for now that biomedicine indeed tends to objectify the human body, for better or worse. However, that objectification is not problematic *in principle* does not rule out that there (a) might be particular instances in which objectification might be detrimental to the patient's recovery and well-being, or (b) that the objectification of the human body might miss out on aspects of health and illness that are relevant to medical practice. This second remark brings me to the second claim justifying the phenomenology of medicine: is biomedicine, insofar as it has health as its object, indeed premised on a flawed ontology of the body?

This question can be answered relatively shortly here if we are willing to accept three premises. The first premise is that—as I have suggested in the introduction—a naturalistic account (e.g., Boorse's biostatistical theory of health) is indeed central in medical practice and structures how health and illness are understood and investigated. Second, we should accept that such a naturalistic account of health and disease can be meaningfully interpreted as leading to a biomedical gaze that results in a particular ontology grounded in the objectification of the body. The third premise consists in accepting the adequacy of phenomenological analyses of embodiment (e.g., the distinction between *Leib* and *Körper*, the understanding of embodiment in terms of an "I can"). Now, *if* we accept these three premises, it is quite evident that biomedicine is incapable of coming to a complete understanding of health. Naturalistic accounts of health conceive of the body as an object that is to be described in terms of physiological processes and treat these processes as having the final word about what a human body is. Clearly, such an understanding of the human body is flawed if we are willing to accept that the objectivity of the human body is not ontologically foundational.

This brings me to the last question: does phenomenology indeed enable to articulate those aspects relevant to health and illness that are typically removed from view in medical practice? The claim of phenomenologists of medicine typically is that phenomenology enables to elucidate the lived experience of health and illness. Let us assume for now that phenomenology can indeed relevantly contribute in this regard. However, from the phenomenological analyses of embodiment discussed in this chapter, it follows that the body's objectivity is crucial as well and that this objectivity often recedes from experience. As Drew Leder puts it: "The phenomenologist of the body is already, and necessarily, a hermeneut. To explore the region of the body most hidden from awareness is merely to extend this hermeneutical approach" (Leder, 1990b, p. 37). But why should we accept that the hermeneutic activities of the phenomenologist should be prioritised over those of medical science (cf. de Boer, 2021; Ihde, 1998)? And why should we accept that phenomenology is the most adequate method to shed light on the *synthesis* of the subjective and objective aspects of the human body?

One way of answering these questions would be to simply say that phenomenology can say relevant things about the lived experience of health and illness and in the end does not make any ontological claims. The main contribution to phenomenology to medicine would then be pragmatic in that it complements medical practice and helps to better centralise the concerns of patient through its focus on lived experiences of health and illness. It is, however, not self-evident that it should be phenomenology that complements the alleged naturalism of biomedicine. As Sholl has argued, *if* the goal of phenomenology of medicine is to centralise the patient's concerns, then it is not clear beforehand why sciences such as psychology are unable to take these into account while remaining in a third-person perspective (Sholl, 2015, p. 400). This problem seems especially urgent since the third-person perspectives of psychology and that of biomedicine might be more naturally integrated, because these different disciplines does not need to bridge the gap between first- and third-person perspectives assumed in phenomenology.

This argument is certainly alluring insofar as phenomenology is conceived of as a pragmatic addition to medical practice. However, if we take phenomenology as offering an ontology of the body—as I do, a merger of psychology and biomedicine is not able to formulate an adequate account of health because it continues to neglect the *Leib*-character of the body, as well as the synthesis between *Leib* and *Körper*. And as we saw earlier in this chapter, these latter terms cannot straightforwardly be equated with the "subjectivity" and "objectivity" of the body. Rather, it is their integration and synthesis that is constitutive of being-in-the-world, already prior to any objectification in a medical context.

Romano traces the idea that any experience of my own body as an object is a modification of original being-in-the-world all the way back to Husserl: "Now, the possibility of a 'double-sensation' in Husserl's sense certainly exists but it belongs to a rather artificial attitude; it is only a *particular*, and moreover a quite *rare* way in which I experience my own embodiment or corporeality" (Romano, 2016, p. 459). Husserl grounds the body's constitution in tactuality that is exemplified by my hands touching each other. He treats this experience as a unique event and a model for the structure of our embodiment. However, as Romano points out, there are many other ways in which I experience my own corporeality (e.g., looking at my body, having my body touched by others, etc.). These other ways occur way more frequent in our ordinary experience, and it is unclear why we should accept that the double-sensation should be understood as an original experience that uniquely grounds embodiment. Now, insofar as phenomenology of medicine criticises biomedicine for not having access to first-person experience because it cannot access an authentic layer of embodiment, it is worthwhile to consider if—accepting Romano's critique of Husserl—it is possible at all to have experiential access to one's bodily constitution.

Leder seems to be acutely aware of this problematic when describing the visceral depths of one's body that escape experiential awareness, yet at the same influence how one understands one's body. He maintains that the objectification of the body does not originate in medical practice, nor is it unique to it: "[T]he sense of the body as an *alien* thing does not arise solely in the objectifications of the modern physician. Prior to visiting the doctor's office, the pain and disability of the patient have already laid the groundwork for a distanced perspective" (Leder, 1990b, p. 77, my emphasis). This implies that the body is constituted in such a way that the interaction between *Leib* and *Körper* is given and not the result of the engagement with a particular kind of practice. The experience of being objectified, therefore, need not be the result of biomedicine.

What is striking in Leder's description of objectification above is that he explicitly states that objectification is accompanied with the sensing of one's body as something *alien* or as Zaner would have it, *uncanny*. While there certainly might be cases—like pain or illness—in which objectification and a sense of alienation coincide; think, for example, how your foot appears when you have stepped into a rusty nail and you have to pull the nail out. However, such alienation does not need to be there in every case of objectification—as if being-in-the-world presupposes a harmony between *Leib* and *Körper* (de Boer, 2020). As Zeiler (2010) has suggested, there are many instances in which one's body is explicitly thematised as an object of attention but does not appear as alien: when looking into the mirror after a round of physical exercises, I perceive my body in terms of an ownness, in terms of the results of the previous exercise.

And even in a doctor's office, the objectification of one's body in pain—both by oneself and from the doctor's third-person perspective—need not result in alienation. As Fuchs puts it:

> The fact that I can state meaningfully: "I have pains in my foot" and can also show the doctor the same foot presupposes that the subjective space of my pain and the objective space of my foot do not belong to two separate worlds [...]. It presupposes *that the subjective and the objective space of my body syntopically coincide.*
>
> (Fuchs, 2018, p. 17)

Again, here we see that the intertwinement of the subjectivity and objectivity of the body is a vehicle that enables the constitution of a shared space in which the body does not appear as a foreign object to either party but as a point of orientation that can be meaningfully interpreted by both parties.

What the above discussion shows is that a phenomenological ontology of the body, even when it might not function as a pragmatic complement to naturalism, cannot be surpassed when one intends to develop an account of health and illness. If one's body is constituted in the relationship between *Leib* and *Körper*, investigating the structure of this relationship is crucial for understanding the constitution of the experience of being healthy or ill.

§1.3 Conclusion: Phenomenology and the Issue of Normality

Phenomenological approaches to health and illness importantly counter approaches that primarily conceive of health and medicine in terms of biomedicine. However, as I have suggested in this chapter, phenomenological analyses of health and illness typically conceive of health as a state in which our bodies are not thematised in experience such that we can engage without problems in our everyday activities. Sholl (2015, p. 401) points out that this suggests that phenomenologists tend to assume a close proximity between health and normality or even simply equate the terms; after all, health is equated with the ability to be able to engage in the *normal* course of things, where the body's transparency is a "hallmark of health and normal function" (Carel, 2008, p. 39).

Above, building on Sholl's argument, I already suggested that there are many occasions in which our body ceases to be transparent that remain part of the experience of being healthy. I argued that not every instance of objectification is a marker of illness, but also that such a claim does not necessarily pose a problem to the phenomenologist. The issue of normality, I believe to touch on a fundamental problem for phenomenological approaches to health and illness though. After all, the embodied subject is not completely free in deciding which experiences fall within the spectrum of the normal. The experience of normality is constituted in relation to both the visceral depths of one's own body and in relation to certain societal and institutional norms. Whereas, in principle, a phenomenological analysis could account for the former relationship, it has difficulties accounting for the latter: the experience of normalcy partly involves what others—from a third-person perspective—perceive to be normal. As we will see in the next two chapters, Foucault's work helps articulating how the experience of health is also socially constituted, and hence is dependent on living in a world that is shared with others.

The lack of attention for how the experience of normalcy—and thereby of health—can be partly explained by the tendency in phenomenology to understand medicine primarily in terms of a "the medical encounter" between doctor and patient. However, the ways in which individuals encounter "the medical" are way more complex than presupposed when taking the doctor-patient relationship as the central unit of medical practice. And this situation is getting even more complex due to an increasing focus on preventive medicine that takes people's lifestyles as a starting point. Because such complexities are often neglected, phenomenologists of medicine tend to conceive too much of the embodied experience of health as being isolated from the socio-cultural background against which they occur. This idea and the accompanied prioritisation of subjective experience as being primary to—or more authentic then—the practice of scientific objectification in medicine problematically presupposes a strict distinction between life in a physiological sense, and life in an existential sense. However, as I will argue in more detail in the next chapter, the experience of health does not only involve a relationship between *Leib* and *Körper* but also with what is considered to be a normal—or healthy—body within the population of which that body is a part.

Addressing this latter relationship requires, so I will suggest, to build a bridge between a phenomenological and a Foucauldian approach to health. The latter approach enables to explain how the "normal" body within a population is constituted and how this normal body has a bearing on the experience of health. For instance, in the 19th century the direct observation of diseased organs became a model for attaining the truth about the body, leading to a quite particular understanding of normalcy and deviancy. Leder tries to read this development in phenomenological terms: "While Foucault addresses this as a historical development, it manifests my phenomenological point; life itself is allied to a certain concealment, a withdrawal and protection of its vital center" (Leder, 1990b, p. 45). Even if life is always allied to a certain concealment, it seems hard to deny that our experience of health is not also constituted by how life is brought into *unconcealment* as a result of particular (institutionalised) practices of objectification. The work of Foucault does not primarily affirm a prior phenomenological truth, but instead, as we will see, helps to rethink the constitution of health and illness beyond the limits of our own bodies.

Notes

1 For example, Carman (1999) maintains that there is a strong discontinuity between Husserl and Merleau-Ponty, whereas Heinämaa (2002) challenges this position. For an overview of Merleau-Ponty's reading of Husserl, see for example: Toadvine & Embree (2002).

2 In this chapter, I do not touch upon questions about Merleau-Ponty's methodology in that I will discuss the reliability of the results of the case-studies (e.g., patient Schneider), nor the adequacy of Merleau-Ponty's interpretation of

them. For an insightful analysis of the use of pathology as a phenomenological method, see Carel (2021).

3 Leder (1990b, pp. 62–68) establishes a link between the invisibility of visceral depth in Merleau-Ponty's analysis of the flesh and the chiasm and in his unfinished and posthumously published book *The Visible and the Invisible* (1968). An in-depth discussion of these concepts is beyond the scope of this chapter, but see for example: de Boer and Verbeek (2022, pp. 192–195).

4 This is not necessarily to say that a strict distinction between health and illness can be made in the absolute. Whether or not something can be qualified as illness is, according to Svenaeus, dependent on the extent to which such an experience gives rise to a long-term alien attunement that prevents a person to project oneself into the future.

References

Burwood, S. (2008). The apparent truth of dualism and the uncanny body. *Phenomenology & the Cognitive Sciences*, 7, 263–278.

Carel, H. (2008). *Illness: The cry of the flesh*. Acumen Publishing.

Carel, H. (2016). *Phenomenology of illness*. Oxford University Press.

Carel, H. (2021). Pathology as a phenomenological tool. *Continental Philosophy Review*, *54*(2), 201–217. https://doi.org/10.1007/s11007-021-09538-9

Carel, H., & Kidd, I.J. (2014). Epistemic injustice in healthcare: A philosophical analysis. *Medicine, Health Care and Philosophy, 17*(4), 529–540. https://doi.org/10.1007/s11019-014-9560-2

Carman, T. (1999). The body in Husserl and Merleau-Ponty. *Philosophical Topics*, *27*(2), 205–226.

de Boer, B. (2020). Experiencing objectified health: Turning the body into an object of attention. *Medicine, Health Care and Philosophy*, *23*, 401–411. https://doi.org/10.1007/s11019-020-09949-0

de Boer, B. (2021). *How scientific instruments speak: Technological mediations in scientific practice*. Lexington Books.

de Boer, B., & Verbeek, P.P-. (2022). Living in the flesh: Technologically mediated chiasmic relationships (in times of a pandemic). *Human Studies*, *45,* 189–208. https://doi.org/10.1007/s10746-022-09625-78

Fuchs, T. (2018). *Ecology of the brain: The phenomenology and biology of the embodied mind*. Oxford University Press.

Gallagher, S. (1986). Body image and body schema: A conceptual clarification. *The Journal of Mind and Behavior*, *7*(4), 541–554.

Heidegger, M. (1985). *Being and time* (J. Macquarrie & E. Robinson, trans.). Basil Blackwell.

Heinämaa, S. (2002). From decisions to passions: Merleau-Ponty's interpretation of Husserl's reduction. In T. Toadvine & L. Embree (Eds.), *Merleau-Ponty's reading of Husserl* (pp. 127–146). Springer.

Husserl, E. (1989). *Ideas pertaining to a pure phenomenology and to a phenomenological philosophy. Second book: Studies in the phenomenology of constitution* (R. Rojcewicz & A. Schuwer). Kluwer.

Ihde, D. (1998). *Expanding hermeneutics: Visualism in science*. Northwestern University Press.

Ihde, D. (2002). *Bodies in technology*. University of Minnesota Press.

Leder, D. (1990a). Flesh and blood: A proposed supplement to Merleau-Ponty. *Human Studies*, *13*, 209–219.

Leder, D. (1990b). *The Absent Body*. The University of Chicago Press.

Merleau-Ponty, M. (1968). *The visible and the invisible* (A. Lingis, trans.). Northwestern University Press.
Merleau-Ponty, M. (2012). *Phenomenology of perception* (D.A. Landes, trans.). Routledge.
Romano, C. (2016). After the lived-body. *Continental Philosophy Review*, *49*, 445–468. https://doi.org/10.1007/s11007-016-9398-9
Slatman, J. (2019). The *Körper-Leib* distinction. In A. Murphy, G. Salamon, & G. Weiss (Eds.), *50 Concepts for a critical phenomenology* (pp. 203–209). Northwestern University Press.
Sholl, J. (2015). Putting phenomenology in its place: Some limits of a phenomenology of medicine. *Theoretical Medicine and Bioethics*, *36*(6), 391–410. https://doi.org/s10.1007/s11017-015-9345-5
Svenaeus, F. (2001). *The hermeneutics of medicine and the phenomenology of health: Steps towards a philosophy of medical practice*. Springer.
Svenaeus, F. (2013). Naturalistic and phenomenological theories of health: Distinctions and connections. *Royal Institute of Philosophy Supplement*, *72*, 221–238. https://doi.org/10.1017/s135824611000l2x
Svenaeus, F. (2019). A defense of the phenomenological account of health and illness. *The Journal of Medicine and Philosophy*, *44*(4), 459–478. https://doi.org/10.1093/jmp/jhz013
Svenaeus, F. (2023). The phenomenology of objectification in and through medical practice and technology development. *The Journal of Medicine and Philosophy*, *48*(2), 141–150. https://doi.org/10.1093/jmp/jhad007
Toadvine, T., & Embree, L. (2002). *Merleau-Ponty's reading of Husserl*. Springer.
Zaner, R.M. (1981). The context of self. *Ohio University Press*.
Zeiler, K. (2010). A phenomenological analysis of bodily self-awareness in the experience of pain and pleasure: On bodily dys-appearance and eu-appearance. *Medicine, Health Care and Philosophy*, *13*, 333–342. https://doi.org/10.1007/s11019-010-9237-4

2 Our Three Bodies

Medicalisation, Population, Public Health

Introduction

> *But do thou row past them, and anoint the ears of thy comrades with sweet wax, which thou hast kneaded, lest any of the rest may hear. But if thou thyself hast a will to listen, let them bind thee in the swift ship hand and foot upright in the step of the mast, and let the ropes be made fast at the ends to the mast itself, that with delight thou mayest listen to the voice of the two Sirens.*
>
> (Homer, *The Odyssey,* 12.45–53)

On the 10-year journey from Troy back to Ithaca, Odysseus and his crew face many cruelties. Amongst them is their encounter with the goddess Circe, who warns Odysseys about future dangers. The first danger on Odysseus' path is the Sirens who attract sailors with their beautiful voices but turn into savage monsters when the sailors come too close. Odysseus desires to enjoy the beautiful voices of the Sirens without running the risk of ending up their victim. To realise this, he asks his crew to tie him to the mast of the ship and to put wax in their ears that block the voices of the Sirens and to prevent them to hear how Odysseus begs the sailors to untie him.

The safety of everyone on board as well as the possibility for Odysseus to enjoy the Siren's song is dependent on a particular sociotechnical configuration that shapes the experience of everyone involved: it involves a particular hierarchical relation between Odysseus and his crew, as well as the presence of certain techniques and materials like wax and ropes. This example from Antiquity indicates that the experience of one's body and the projects that one can engage in take shape in relation to the projects that others wish to engage in. Furthermore, it indicates that embodiment reflects pre-existing social structures; after all, in the example of the Sirens, it is Odysseus who ends up constraining his body so that he can enjoy the voices of the Sirens, whereas the bodies of the boatmen must attain a different shape for the journey to continue.

DOI: 10.4324/9781003602385-3

I would like to infer from this example that the phenomenological distinction between *Leib* and *Körper* as applied in the context of health that was discussed in the previous chapter, insufficiently recognises how bodies take shape in relation to the bodies of others. This is a crucial omission, since the experience of health does not occur in isolation but is one that is collectively shaped. We cannot evade being part of a social and institutional context that in one way or another prescribes what should be considered healthy, provides norms about what constitutes a healthy body, and which activities we should engage in to stay healthy.

Moreover, the current norms around health and illness are heavily informed by what Foucault calls the clinical or medical gaze, as well as by more recent developments in molecular biology that enable to visualise vital processes taking place inside the body. Phenomenological analyses of health tend to conceive of such norms as potentially unwanted intruders into people's own experiences of health and embodiment and tend to stress that the embodied experience of health should be celebrated as a counterweight against the overly cold gaze of the biomedical sciences (e.g., Carel, 2016; Svenaeus, 2001; Toombs, 1992). While phenomenological discussions of health indeed enable to develop an important critique on the monopoly of the biomedical gaze, it can be questioned if they can give a sufficient description of healthy embodiment without taking into account how the experience of health is shaped by social and biomedical norms.

It is the goal of this chapter to reveal how societal norms, institutional concerns and public health goals are an integral part of the experience of health. As I will argue, this is not the case because they are external forces that exercise power on the body from the outside, but instead because they actively constitute what one's body is, and hence co-shape the experience of healthy embodiment. In doing so, my aim is not to leave phenomenology behind and argue that its focus on the first-person experience of being healthy is flawed. Instead, my suggestion is that a focus on the social and institutional norms around health allows for giving a richer description and enlarged understanding of what the experience of healthy embodiment consists in.

The chapter is structured as follows: first, I introduce the notion of medicalisation and the way it can be used to critique a "healthism" present in many societies. The work of Ivan Illich will be used to exemplify this critique. Second, I suggest that one of the key problems in Illich's analysis is his premise that it is possible to make a distinction between medical and cultural-symbolic norms such that the importance—or authenticity—of the latter can be emphasised. Third, on the basis of Foucault's work—and his critique of Illich—I argue that, precisely because we indeed live in a medicalised society, it is not possible to take recourse to extra-medical norms when developing a concept of health. Instead, I suggest, since medicalisation is grounded in a particular constitution of one's body as being part of a population that is to be governed, the embodied experience of being healthy inescapably ties in with an ontology of the body as part of a population.

§2.1 The Medicalisation Critique

Sophocles' play *Philoctetes* depicts the tragic fate of the Greek (anti-) hero Philoctetes in the Greek war against Troy. In this play, Odysseus and Neoptolemus (Achilles' son) visit the island of Lemnos in search of Philoctetes, or better, of his bow. This is because prophecy has stated that Troy would not fall without the involvement of Philoctetes' bow. Before going to Troy, Philoctetes was one of the great heroes of the Greeks and known as a great archer. However, during the journey to Troy, he was bit in his leg by a snake, which caused a painful wound. Not only that, also the wound was disgusting to see and smelt horrendously. Philoctetes, because he was in pain, screamed during the nights, keeping awake the other Greek warriors. These warriors (including Odysseus) could stand neither the smell of the wound nor Philoctetes' screams, so they guiled Philoctetes into waiting for their (short) return on the desolated island of Lemnos. The Greeks did not come back for ten years and only regained interest in Philoctetes when the prophecy about his bow was revealed. The plot of the play revolves around the issue of whether to betray Philoctetes' again by stealing his bow and leaving him to die on the desolated island, or to recognise him as a hurting individual in need of care.

Philoctetes' story contains several elements that are relevant to the purposes of this chapter. First, it highlights how being part of a certain collective—or social body—crucially forms the experience of being healthy or ill in terms of the individual's ability to form projects. Second, it shows that the visibility of illness does not necessarily culminate in a collective desire to cure it, but can instead also give rise to the exclusion of the sick individual from the collective of which it is a part (Leder, 1990). Third, it indicates that the collective in question that eventually decides on the abandonment of an individual does itself not necessarily benefit from this act.

One crucial difference between Sophocles' play and the current societal focus on health is that whereas Philoctetes was visibly ill and his illness could be clearly linked to an earlier cause (the snakebite), current public health measures intend to prevent illness from taking place before any recognisable (visual) markers are present. Furthermore, there is an important difference in terms of the institutionalisation of health issues, which has greatly increased the quantity in which judgements about one's health status affect one's capacities of action.

The profound influence of health norms on our everyday lives and the role of the biomedical sciences and healthcare institutions in providing and managing health have been extensively analysed within philosophy and sociology alike, giving rise to the widespread idea that our lives have become increasingly *medicalised*. Peter Conrad, one of the most important sociologists studying medicalisation, provides the following definition: X is medicalised when "defined in medical terms, described using medical language, understood through the adoption of a medical framework, or 'treated' with a medical intervention" (Conrad, 2007, p. 5).[1] The typical focus of medicalisation studies is on problems and issues that have only become recently medicalised, or of which it is not immediately obvious that they *should* be medicalised. The goal of studying such cases, then, is to unravel the processes through which these phenomena have become medicalised and which interests are being served in doing so.

In principle, the notion of medicalisation is a neutral or descriptive one, but in practice it has primarily been used to be critical of the increasingly large role of medicine in our daily lives (Conrad, 2007; Wardrope, 2015). In its most extreme form, medicalisation is being criticised for having an adverse effect on the health of individuals. According to the social critic Ivan Illich, for example, medicalisation actively makes people sick: "[W]hat has turned health care into a sick-making enterprise is the very intensity of an engineering endeavor that has translated human survival from the performance of organisms into the result of technical manipulation" (Illich, 1976, p. 7). In similar vein, others have conceived of medicalisation in terms of medicine's overstepping of its legitimate boundaries, leading to a situation in which it has become able to exercise too much power on the everyday lives of individuals (e.g., Rose, 2007a). According to some, the increase in power over the everyday lives of individuals is the result of a particular form of medicalisation, namely *bio*medicalisation (e.g., Clarke & Shim, 2011).[2] This form of medicalisation is considered to be especially pervasive (1) because it focuses on the individual's lifestyle and its relevance to health, thereby potentially turning one's lifestyle into an object of governance that should be strictly monitored in relation to certain health norms, and (2) because it is closely connected to the financial interests of corporations that develop all kinds of products to contribute to lifestyle governance. In both cases, medicalisation implies the illegitimate of power to medical institutions or corporate actors in the medical sphere, which goes at the expense of the power of individuals over their lives, which eventually has a negative effect on health.

§2.1.1 *Medical Nemesis*

Ivan Illich's position as developed in *Medical Nemesis* is a good example of a critical perspective on medicalisation. The first sentence of his book crudely summarises his view: "The medical establishment has become a major threat to health" (Illich, 1976, p. 3). In our modern times, so he maintains, a novel epidemic of disease has spread, which he terms *Iatrogenesis*: an epidemic that originates in the activities of doctors and physicians. According to Illich, this epidemic gives rise to what he calls the *Medical Nemesis*: "By transforming pain, illness, and death from a personal challenge into a technical problem, medical practice expropriates the potential of people to deal with their human condition in an autonomous way and becomes the source of a new kind of un-health" (Illich, 2003, p. 919). Assessing the credibility of this view requires answering the questions: what does Illich take health to be? And how can it be threatened by the very institutions that claim to have a positive effect on health and have been remarkably successful in treating many diseases that were not treatable before, and have greatly expanded the average lifespan of individuals?

The starting point of Illich's critique resembles that of the phenomenologists of medicine: a key issue is that health is nowadays often understood as an entity that can be objectified and scrutinised from a third-person perspective. Obtaining knowledge of health requires obtaining knowledge of physiological or molecular processes taking place inside one's body, which crucially relies on the expertise of medical professionals. The naturalist view defended by Christopher Boorse, discussed in the introduction, is a good example of this account of health. On such accounts, health appears first and foremost as a scientific object that can be isolated and systematically investigated by means of biomedical techniques. For Illich, by contrast, health is not an observable object that falls within the domain of medicine but instead "simply [is] an everyday word that is used to designate the intensity with which individuals cope with their internal states and their environmental conditions" (Illich, 1976, p .7). Hence, health is a particular way in which individuals relate to both themselves and the environment. Instead of a specific identifiable object, health appears here as a way of coping that needs to be cultivated.

For Illich, the capacity of coping is crucial to health because the experiences of pain, sickness and death are an integral part of human life (Illich, 2003, p. 922). Health, then, designates the capacity to cope with those elements of life that provoke struggle and which make it that life does not appear as self-evident. Being able to do so presupposes that individuals have a degree of autonomy and freedom in how they respond to the challenges that life poses. As Illich puts it: "health designates the range of autonomy within which a person exercises control over his own biological states and over the conditions of his immediate environment" (Illich, 1976, p. 242). Since humans inevitably have to relate to both their environment and their own mortality, they are never *completely* free in how to cope with the challenges of life. However, Illich assumes that there is some kind of natural coping mechanism that makes it possible to relate to the challenges that individuals have not chosen themselves, and that autonomy is a condition for responding adequately to such challenges and allows to integrate them into one's life.

Health is, for Illich, not only a capacity to exercise control, but also a right that individuals should have. Health inevitably depends on the environmental circumstances that people inhabit, which makes that it is partly a political question, since the capacity of coping "depends on the way in which political actions condition the milieu and create those circumstances that favour self-reliance, autonomy and dignity for all, particularly the weaker. In consequence, health levels will be at their optimum when the environment brings out autonomous personal, responsible coping ability" (Illich, 1976, p. 7). Insofar as health is a right, it thus becomes a political task to create those kinds of environments that facilitate freedom and autonomous decision-making, as well as cultivate the capacity to cope with the inevitable challenges of human life.

Whereas Illich repeatedly stresses the importance of autonomy for health, he does not conceive of autonomy as a capacity that individuals can exercise in splendid isolation. As we saw already, life always involves a relationship with both the environment and a certain bodily configuration that one has not chosen. Additionally, however, Illich also takes health to be something that takes shape differently in different cultures. He goes even as far to say that "to a large extent culture and health coincide" (Illich, 1976, p. 128). This is because each culture embodies a specific set of attitudes towards pain, disease, death, ageing, impairment, etc. These attitudes are materialised in habits, customs and rituals that embody a particular way of taking up the challenges of life and help to develop a way of coping with them.

For Illich, health consists of the capacity of coping autonomously with the challenges of life, as well as the creation or sustainment of those environments and cultures that actively contribute to autonomous coping. One could say that, given the increase in access to healthcare facilities and the increase in average lifespan, political actions have greatly contributed to the creation of a more favourable environment in the past two centuries, and have contributed to the development of a specific culture in which the challenges of life attain a specific place. However, from the perspective of Illich, the medicalised environment undermines the capacity of autonomous coping, as individuals are only allowed to come to terms with the challenges of life by asking the biomedical sciences for answers, which deprives them of a natural mechanism that helps to deal with the inevitable sufferings of human life. Because of this, "health has ceased to be a native endowment each human being is presumed to possess until proven ill, and has become an ever-receding goal to which one is entitled by virtue of social justice" (Illich, 1976, p. 122). As I will discuss in detail below, he takes medicalisation to undermine both of these aspects: medicalisation undermines autonomous decision-making by incorporating increasingly many aspects of human life into a medical regime. Additionally, medicalisation prevents the creation of those environments and cultures that support autonomous coping, but should rather be seen as creating a non-culture in which the inevitable sufferings of life can no longer be adequately faced.

§2.1.2 *Medicalisation as Iatrogenesis*

To understand Illich's assessment of modern medicine, it is necessary to discuss in more detail why he holds that it undermines human autonomy and contributes to the development of a non-culture. Illich's point is not primarily that every form of medical treatment should be avoided and is necessarily adverse to health. Rather, he holds that medicalisation should be understood as iatrogenesis because it embodies what he calls a *specific counterproductivity*. Whereas the treatment of people clearly can be beneficial to health and medicine can be an integral part of it, iatrogenesis emerges when the system of treatment reaches a certain tipping point which makes it run counter to the initial aims (e.g., caring for the health of people) that it had initially set (Illich, 1976, p. 8). According to Illich, this tipping point has been reached in 20th-century medicine, which is why he holds that the medical establishment has become a threat to health and constitutes the epidemic of iatrogenesis.

Illich distinguishes between three ways in which the medical establishment undermines health: (1) clinical iatrogenesis, (2) social iatrogenesis and (3) cultural iatrogenesis. *Clinical iatrogenesis* refers to the therapeutic side effects of medical treatment, such as infections by hospital bacteria, or the side effects of drugs used to treat a specific problem. In itself, this form of iatrogenesis is not unique to 20th-century medicine. However, it has been intensified because of the increase in medicine's power and according increase in the use of pharmaceutical drugs, as well as in clinical interventions (Illich, 1976, p. 27).

Social iatrogenesis designates those impairments to health that are due to the socio-economic transformations instantiated by the institutionalisation of health care. It indicates that every experience of suffering is only recognised as such when it is medically acknowledged. This, in turn, might induce additional stress in individuals, as well as gives rise to a tendency to expect immediate medical treatment for almost every form of intolerance (Illich, 1976, p. 41). Hence, social iatrogenesis undermines health, because it constitutes a situation in which every form of suffering is considered to be unhealthy or deviant, and only takes seriously those forms of suffering that have been incorporated within a medical regime.[3]

Cultural iatrogenesis is, for Illich, the most crucial dimension of medical health-denial, as it "saps the will of people to suffer their reality" (Illich, 1976, p. 127). In a medicalised society, every form of suffering appears as unnecessary and treatable, instead of being an intricate part of human life. In doing so, the medical enterprise explicitly or implicitly denounces other cultural habits and practices to deal with suffering as being unimportant are not sufficiently credible. Whereas, according to Illich, these socio-cultural habits and practices allow for developing a subjective or intersubjective understanding of the reality of human life that inevitably involves suffering and helps developing an autonomous coping mechanism with regard to life, a medicalised society prevents the development of such an understanding and hence of any possibility of autonomous coping.

It is not possible to evade iatrogenesis as an individual, because of the power that medical institutions exercise. As Illich puts it: "In every society, medicine, like law and religion, defines what is normal, proper, desirable. Medicine has the authority to label one man's complains a legitimate illness, to declare a second man sick though he himself does not complain, and to refuse a third social recognition of his pain, his disability and even his death" (Illich, 1976, p. 45). The authority of medicine and the power that comes from it puts forward a structure of normality that individuals need to submit to in order to remain participating in society. This exercise of power undermines the potentiality of individuals to exercise their own power and act autonomously when determining what constitutes normal and non-normal aspects of their lives.

The medical legitimation of the exercise of power is the underlying conception of the human body as a machine and its health as being subject to mechanical laws. Investigating the body and its health status leads to the equation of medicine and engineering. To carry out one's role of doctor or healthcare professional best requires to act as a master-engineer that observes a machine-like body and intervenes when the threat of malfunctioning becomes visible. The appropriate response to decay and suffering is, from an engineering point of view, to engage in the ongoing management of the body from an external point of view.

According to Illich, it is this perception of the body that implicitly—but not legitimately—justifies the power that medicine exercises in society. Viewing the body in this way gives rise to a very specific conception of medicine; one that does not so much focus on suffering, but rather on sickness understood as the malfunctioning of the bodily machine (Illich, 1976, p. 160). Furthermore, individual bodies are understood as being part of a larger machine—society—that must remain functioning. As I will clarify in more detail in the next sections, this makes the needs of individuals subordinate to the needs of a larger whole of which they are part, such that individual autonomy appears as a hindrance to the attempt to maintain and preserve society as a whole. As a result of this development, so Illich posits, medicine will remain to exercise increasingly more power on individuals because the maintenance of the whole will create a situation in which "preventive procedures become compulsory, and the right of the patient to withhold consent to his own treatment vanishes as the doctor argues that he must submit to diagnosis, since society cannot afford the burden of curative procedures that would be even more expensive" (Illich, 1976, p. 97).

The power that medicine exercises and the decrease in the ability of autonomous coping that it institutes are thus justified with reference to the "health" of a particular societal organisation that must be preserved. For this reason, the individual right to health becomes increasingly important. This situation can only be changed, so Illich holds, by a restructuring of the societal organisation that is grounded in a different perception of what a body is, which is why he takes the issue of health and the countering of medicalisation to be a political project eventually. Illich juxtaposes a non-medicalised social organisation with the medicalisation of life that is demanded by a particular form of organisation starting in the 20th century, and urges politics to reform medical institutions and to a certain extent return to pre-medicalised societies or cultures. Medicalisation forms a threat to health because it keeps existing societal structures in place and actively defends their ongoing existence at the cost of the individual's capacity to face the sufferings that belong to life autonomously and give them a proper place.

§2.2 From Individual Health to Public Health

Illich problematises modern medicine because it conceives of the body as a purely material object that can be manipulated at will, and that *should* be manipulated in particular ways for a particular societal organisation to be preserved. As a result, medicine has fundamentally overstepped its boundaries and has turned itself from something that can assist in facing human suffering into a threat to health that is laden with political and ideological assumptions about normality. As I indicated in the introduction, utterances such as "smoking is bad for your health" turn health into a moral obligation by questioning if smoking is a habit that can be exercised by a "good person" (Metzl, 2010). Other examples are the economic interests of app-developing companies for promoting self-tracking applications as being beneficial for one's health, or the political interests when promoting same-sex marriages as the healthy norm. In each of these cases, it is clear that the notion of health used is far from value-free but rather is part of a normative discourse that helps constituting what is "normal".

As we saw, Illich condemns such discourses as suppressing more authentic ways of coping with the challenges of life and urges us to develop our own norms and coping mechanisms. This leads to a complete rejection of medicalisation as producing the wrong norms, in that the norms it produces are adverse to living a healthy life.

A clear distinction between symbolic or cultural practices and norms and those of medicine seems to underlie Illich's rejection: medical norms are excluded from the cultural practices that allegedly enable people to cope with life's inevitable sufferings. At the same time, it has been questioned if this distinction between the symbolic/cultural and the medical can currently be maintained—or even if it has ever been possible to make this distinction. If symbolic or cultural norms and medical norms are intertwined, should we not acknowledge that both biomedicine and public health "may be viewed as contributing to the moral regulation of society, focusing as they do upon ethical and moral practices of the self" (Lupton, 1995, p. 4)? Questioning medicalisation should, if we are correct to assume that a clear distinction between medical and cultural norms is impossible, not culminate into a complete rejection of the former norms but instead prompt us to investigate how the two are intertwined and what are the consequences of this intertwinement for one's experience of health.

Lupton's book, *The Imperative of Health* offers an interesting starting point for the latter way of questioning medicalisation. This for two reasons: firstly, it helps clarifying the relationship between biomedicine as a medical practice and the practice of public health, and secondly because it enables to elucidate in what sense medical and symbolic/cultural norms are intertwined by leading us to the work of Michel Foucault. Lupton defines the aim of her book as follows: "What needs to be brought to light and critically interrogated are the covert political and symbolic dimensions of [health] institutions" (1995, p. 5). The idea underlying this aim is that health-related practices cannot be simply equated with interactions between doctors and patients in a hospital setting or in the room of a general practitioner. That is, the objectifying view of the human body is not only to be found in particular settings in which objectification might be justifiable with reference to the goals of medical interventions, but extends, according to Lupton, to the everyday lives of citizens. She identifies public health and health promotion as those practices that are concerned with regulating the health status of larger populations.

The key difference between biomedicine (narrowly understood as those health-related practices taking place in a regulated hospital setting) and public health is, following Lupton, that they are concerned with different objects. The former's object is the body of an individual patient that can be healthy or diseased and can be surgically or pharmaceutically intervened upon, whereas the latter's object is a population that can be described as healthy, as developing normally, or as at risk (Lupton, 1995, p. 4). Typical issues of concern for public health officials and institutions are problems like dirt, poor water supplies, dangerous housing, malnutrition, lifespan or birth control. Each of those problems cannot be clearly traced back to individual bodies that function in a "deficient" manner, but instead must be addressed on the level of a certain collective of bodies: a population. Doing so requires focusing on both adjustments of the environment (e.g., building houses that conform to certain standards) and the behaviour of individuals (e.g., encouraging people to wash their hands or brush their teeth on a regular basis).

But on the basis of what criteria is it possible to determine to which standards houses should conform or how often people should wash their hands? Determining such criteria presupposes to have an idea of what constitutes a "normal" population. Often, such criteria are legitimated with reference to the objectivity and neutrality of the biomedical sciences. However, even if we accept that biomedicine is capable of objectively determining the mechanisms underlying certain diseases, it is more difficult to straightforwardly accept that it can give a univocal answer to the question of what is a normal lifespan or what is the normal amount of children to have. Put differently, convincing someone that biomedicine would be able to do so requires to explain how its claims about individual bodies can be extended to the body of a population, as well as to explain the relationship between the two.

The work of Foucault is relevant for explaining the conditions of possibility of this extension and to highlight in what sense medical norms and symbolic-cultural norms are intertwined in the context of public health. Three interrelated questions are at stake here: (1) which assumptions about the relation between individual and society underlie the extension of biomedicine to the domain of public health?, (2) how do these assumptions inform what constitutes a normal population? and (3) how does it become possible to regulate the behaviour of a population such that it conforms to the norms set upon it?

As I will show in the next sections, Foucault offers a good starting point for answering these questions by interpreting public health—and biomedicine more generally—as an activity that approaches bodies in terms of the population that they are a part (e.g., Foucault, 1978, 1980). The institution of medicine introduces a particular politics of the body by instantiating specific regimes of control that individuals are necessarily involved in. As we will see, this analysis offers a more nuanced picture of how medical norms shape societal and individual behaviour than Illich's analysis discussed above, because Foucault does not assume that it is possible to speak about cultural practices around autonomy and authenticity that are in principle uncontaminated and in need of protection from the demon of a medical nemesis.[4]

§2.3 Foucault and the Conditions of Possibility for Medicalisation: Governing Finitude

The examples of Odysseus and Philoctetes at the beginning of this chapter served to suggest that it is impossible to conceive of the experiences of health and illness independent of the social relations in which they are embedded. While these examples enable to question phenomenological analyses of health and illness insofar the latter tend to substantialise subjective experiences and isolate them from the larger social context in which they occur (cf. Kusters, 2023), they have no direct bearing on the issue of medicalisation. After all, both Odysseus and Philoctetes are not "defined in medical terms, described using medical language, understood through the adoption of a medical framework, or 'treated' with a medical intervention" (Conrad, 2007, p. 5). In this section, I intend to show that a particular conception of the body is a condition of possibility for medicalisation.

Foucault's 1974 lecture, "The crisis of medicine or the crisis of antimedicine" offers a good entry point for studying the conception of the human body presupposed in medicalisation. In this lecture, which can be partly understood as a response to Illich's critique of medicine, Foucault argues that, the 20th century marked the birth of a *somatocracy*: "a regime that sees the care of the body, corporal health, the relation between illness and health, etc. as appropriate areas of State intervention" (Foucault, 2004, p. 7). It is specific to 20th-century regimes to not to consider the soul or the mind as entities that should be taken care of by governmental bodies, but instead, one's body and its health status becomes an object of governmental intervention.

For Foucault's explanation of the process leading up to the emergence of a somatocracy, we must consult two other works: *The Birth of the Clinic* and the essay "The politics of health in the eighteenth century". From these works, three crucial moments for the medicalisation of the body can be identified: (1) the transformation of death from something transcendent into an immanent process, (2) the constitution of a social body (population) that can be controlled and (3) a focus on the family as a unit of control.

In *The Birth of the Clinic*, Foucault argues that the 19th century marked a shift in understanding the relationship between death and life.[5] Death was no longer understood as a transcendent ending-point of human life, indicating a clear break with the natural (i.e., life). Instead, death started to be viewed as a *natural result* of the *natural processes* taking place within the human organism. In Foucault's terms: "It is when death became the concrete a priori of medical experience that death could detach itself from counter-nature and become *embodied* in the *living bodies* of individuals" (Foucault, 2003, p. 196). When death was made immanent, it became possible for doctors to systematically investigate the processes leading to the deterioration of the organism. As a consequence, the human body was constituted as a medical object of which it could be retrospectively identified how it died (e.g., by rendering certain processes pathological), making it possible to observe the pathologies that are potentially harmful to the human organism and to intervene into those. As a result, "[d]eath left its old tragic heaven and became the lyrical core of man: his invisible truth, his visible secret" (Foucault, 2003, p. 172).

The making immanent of death gave rise to a clear medical criterion for distinguishing the "healthy" from the "unhealthy": processes that quicken the occurrence can be called "unhealthy", while processes that are normal and keep death at bay can be called "healthy". As a result, death becomes visibly present as a limit on life, that is yet visible, can be anticipated, and that can be delayed through medical intervention: "[I]n [medicine], death is endlessly repeated, but it is also exorcised; and although it ceaselessly reminds man of the limit that he bears within him, it also speaks to him of that technical world that is the armed, positive, full form of his finitude" (Foucault, 2003, p. 198).

Understanding death, from this point of view, is to understand what are the "normal" processes leading to death, and the circumstances under which death "normally" occurs (Canguilhem, 1991). Making such processes visible presupposes to approach the body as a medical object: the visible secret that is simultaneously the truth of human existence can only be unraveled by means of a medical gaze. The conception of the body underlying this approach is not the lived body of an individual, but a universal objectified body consisting of a set of physiological processes that can be rendered normal or pathological. Making this distinction and being able to develop a relevant understanding of life, then, presupposes that life must be objectified and can only be investigated from an external third-person perspective.

A second development leading up to the birth of the somatocracy was that the making immanent of death was not only applied to individual bodies but to collectives of bodies too. The emergence of the human body as a medical object was accompanied with idea that the human body is part of a larger population—or of a larger "social body" (Foucault, 2004, p. 117). According to Foucault, the "social body" is the body of the population of a certain state, whose health status *as a population* became an object of governmental concern. For states to remain to exist, it is a necessity that their population remains maintained (i.e., that it has a "normal" finitude).

Not only was a population understood in terms of the number of individuals inhabiting a particular area, "but equally in the sense of an ensemble of individuals having between them relations of coexistence and constituting therefore a specific reality" (Foucault, 2014, p. 117). Approaching human bodies in terms of a population presupposes the determination of certain averages relevant to its finitude (e.g., birth rate, death rate, lifespan, disease rates), which can be considered desirable or undesirable. Making such determinations possible requires that governmental institutions gather relevant information from their citizens. On the basis of such information it can for instance be determined what is considered to be an average disease rate. In cases of deviation (e.g., when a disease rate is high in a given area and/or group), governments can start to collect data that enables to explain deviations and to intervene when necessary. For instance, a low birth rate might correlate with certain housing conditions, water quality, general hygiene, etc. This is why Foucault can state that the development of a collective body *as a population* constitutes a new reality: to govern finitude implies to understand and govern the relationships between individuals and between individuals and the environment in terms of factors relevant to the finitude of a given population.

Statistics are crucial for determining the processes relevant to the governance of finitude and make it possible to think of phenomena like death rates as having a particular distribution in a given area. If there is a higher amount of death rates at a particular location—an *abnormality*, with the result that other circumstances at this particular location can become considered to be abnormalities as well. The behaviour of individuals living at a certain location or the environmental circumstances in which they live, then, are factors that appear as being in need of governance in light of the finitude of a population. For instance, when making a link between hygiene and disease rates, it must be ensured that people do engage in behaviours and/or live in environments that conform to certain hygiene standards. These behaviours and environments, hence, became medical objects that are integrated into the governance of finitude.

A third relevant factor in the development of a somatocracy is the constitution of the family as an object of governmental control. Managing the relationship between birth rates and death rates requires, at least, to ensure that (1) a sufficient number of children are born, (2) that a sufficient number of children reach adulthood and (3) that the children reaching adulthood become "healthy" adults. This implies that the relationship between parents and their children must become codified in accordance with specific rules safeguarding that children indeed turn into "healthy" adults (Foucault, 2014, p. 118). Whereas earlier it had been possible to interpret the family in terms of the sphere of the *oikos* that is—or should be—exempt from governmental control, or in terms of a natural process in which children simply inherit certain qualities from their parents, the new politics of health constituted the family as a unit that both falls within the sphere of the government and which cannot be let run its natural course: "It had to become a dense, saturated, permanent and continuous physical environment that surrounded, maintained and promoted the child's body" (Foucault, 2014, p. 118).

Since the relationships within and between families are situated within the larger social body of the population, they are part of the governance of finitude. The relationship(s) between parents and their children should be "optimised" in view of the goal of the health of the larger social body. And since the development of healthy children is key to the maintenance of a healthy social body, the health status of children started to be considered as the main objective of family life. In other words, when the population was constituted as a medical object that can be interpreted in terms of normality and pathology, families simultaneously were medicalised in that their internal dynamics are linked to the development of the population at large. The result of this is a system of collective social control in which parents and their children have the obligation to conform to certain hygiene standards, turn to the appropriate scientific professionals in case of illness: the medicalisation of the family constituted a specific ethic of good health relative to the health of the social body of which it is a part.

§2.3.1 *Foucault and the Medical Nemesis*

With the above genealogy of the somatocracy in mind, we are better able to position Foucault vis-à-vis Illich. Foucault criticises Illich for insufficiently recognising the transformation from medicine into a scientific discipline and the extension of the scope of medicine beyond the wishes of the sick who visit the doctor for help (i.e., the development from medicine into public health). For Foucault, what is specific to modern medicine is not so much that it oversteps its boundaries or undermines more authentic ways of coping with human suffering, but instead what he calls (1) positive iatrogenicity and (2) undefined medicalisation.

Illich uses the term iatrogenesis to express the idea that 20th-century medicine has been the cause of an epidemic of diseases that are the result of the actions of doctors and medical institutions. By introducing the term "positive iatrogenecity", Foucault intends to challenge Illich's claim that 20th century marks the birth of *clinical iatrogenesis*. Medicine certainly can be responsible for the death of individuals—it has the capacity to kill, but this is far from unique to the 20th century. Such deaths used to be attributed to the ignorance of individual doctors or to the fact that medicine could not be considered a true science. However, the 20th century marked a moment in which medicine itself became dangerous, not because it could not rely on certain knowledge or because of individual non-scientific ignorance, but in virtue of its reliance on scientific methods (Foucault, 2004, p. 9).

Foucault defines positive iatrogenicity as "the harmful effects of medication due [...] to the action of medical practice itself, in so far as it has a rational basis" (Foucault, 2004, p. 10). This form of iatrogenicity is not marked by the absence of knowledge of the consequences of particular medical therapy but instead by the fact that those consequences can be estimated but are not exactly known. For instance, anti-infectious treatments are highly successful in combating particular hostile agents but also lead to a decrease in the organism's sensitivity to hostile agents in general. Such negative effects, while known in general, are difficult to evaluate on the level of individual organisms, which is why medical treatment inevitably involves certain unknown risks. The crux, for Foucault, is that what is particular to 20th-century medicine is not that it has the capacity to kill, but rather that it is aware of the harm that it can do and must continuously determine risks by weighing the positive effects of treatments against the negative ones.[6]

One of Illich's critiques of 20th-century medicine is that it has overstepped its boundaries by no longer solely focusing on patients and their individual malaise and by addressing themes beyond the patient's wishes (Foucault, 2004, p. 12). Foucault's disagreement with Illich, here, does not so much concern the fact that the latter's analysis is incorrect but rather that it is grounded in a naiveté about the domains that are already medicalised. Since medicine has evolved into the governance of a population, many aspects of daily life ranging from housing conditions to diets and from sexual behaviour to hygiene, have become themes of concern for medicine. When Illich proposes to (re)turn to a demedicalised practice of health focusing on lifestyle, diet, housing conditions and the like, he fails, according to Foucault, to recognise that those aspects of life are medicalised already:

> But what is hygiene at present except a series of rules set in place and codified by biological and medical knowledge, when it is not medical authority itself that has elaborated it? Anti-medicine can only oppose medicine with facts or projects that have been already set up by certain type of medicine.
>
> (Foucault, 2004, p. 14)

The point being that since the 18th century that marked the start of the governance of the population, any theme in everyday life has the potential to be transformed into a medical theme. This is what, according to Foucault, makes medicalisation *undefined*: there is no—and has never been—a clearly circumscribable area that can be denoted as "medical" and can be opposed to domains that are "non-medical". And the hopes of Illich of taking care of health by supposedly extra-medical means such as cultural practices related to lifestyle and diet are in vain because these health-related practices have been part and parcel of medicalisation since its outset. As Lupton puts it: "Most social issues have become subsumed under the rubric of health, and therefore have been rendered appropriate problems for health promotional intervention" (Lupton, 1995, p. 51). This, in turn, makes it impossible to return to pre-medical—allegedly authentic—practices of care that enable to deal differently with the sufferings necessarily present in life: the issue is not to either be in favour of medicine or against it (as Illich seems to be) but instead to start to understand how themes relevant to the population body are governed and which type of body is perceived as being "normal" and which as deviant.

§2.4 Conclusion: Our Three Bodies

The above responses to Illich, if plausible, indicate that rather than attempting to eliminate the relationships between individuals and the populations of which they are a part, it should be recognised that one's body and its health cannot be cut loose from such governmental attempts. But if there is no possibility to return to a pre-medicalised state in which care can be practised and health can be pursued in response to the medical nemesis, what would be a response inspired by a Foucauldian framework? Must it simply be conceded that increasingly many aspects of life become subsumed under the domain of medicine and are brought outside of our control, such that people become normalised in a particular manner under medicine's authority? The analysis in this chapter has left such questions unanswered because it has not focused on the notion of "power", and how—and to what extent—the government of the population and the constitution of one's body as being part of the population are wound up in power relations.

Before addressing this issue in the next chapter, let us first collect what is gained by addressing the medicalisation through discussing Illich's work and Foucault's response to it. For Foucault, Illich's analysis is grounded in a distinction between a private medicine and an institutionalised medicine. He asks:

> A private, "liberal" medicine, sought out by individual initiative and subject to the mechanisms of supply and demand—and to its side, or perhaps facing it, a medical management determined by the authorities, supported by an administrative apparatus, framed by strict legislative structure, and addressing itself to the entire collectivity. Is it productive to demarcate a clear opposition and to determine which of these two types of medicine was the first, from which the other was derived?
>
> (Foucault, 2014, p. 113)

On the basis of the above analysis, we can conclude that the question posed here is to be understood rhetorically and that it is impossible to clearly distinguish between private and institutionalised medicine. Rather, what Foucault shows is that every experience of health and illness makes in some sense reference to the collective pursuit of medicine. The 18th century marks a shift here, not because it was the time when medicine lost its "private character", but because it produced a new type of administration around the medical body and started to understand "health" as a stand-in for "good health" and as a goal worthy of pursuit. As Lupton puts it, from this moment onwards "'health' therefore denotes more than a medical condition, disease or lack thereof, but comprises a group of knowledges used to assess different populations for different governmental strategies" (Lupton, 1995, p. 70).

This insight has consequences for understanding the body's ontology and complicates the Leib-Körper distinction prevalent in phenomenology. For, insofar as governmental strategies target the bodies of individuals, they do so as them being part of a larger population and not only in terms of them being individual bodies. As a result, it is appropriate to speak about *three* aspects of the body instead of two: *Leib*, *Körper*, and *one's body as part of a population.* The constitution of the body, therefore, involves the institutional and governmental health context in which it is situated. Whereas *Körper* involves the objectification of an individual body within a particular medical context, the body as part of a population explicitly objectifies the individual body in relation to the reference frame of the population of which it is a part. The experience of one's body *as a* body that is part of a population might give rise to particular experiences of health and illness, normality and abnormality. This indicates that one's body in its health status are constituted in relation to a shared standard of normality and presupposes the existence of a shared world that is governed in a particular way.

The question then becomes, and this is the question to be addressed in the next chapter, if governmental control and the power that governments exercise in the end have the final say in distinguishing between health and illness, between normal and abnormal. That is, does the objectifying power of governmental control eventually determine how individuals experience their own body as a healthy body? Or is there a possibility to have experiences of health that are not institutionally determined?

Notes

1 While Conrad's definition of medicalisation is influential, a wide range of other definitions can be found in the literature. In this chapter, I will primarily rely on Conrad's definition and only intend to highlight that the notion can be used both descriptively and critically. In either case, the fact that increasingly many phenomena have become medicalised supports my argument that the embodied experience of health is inevitably collective and institutionally shaped. For an

overview of different definitions of medicalisation, see for instance, Hoffmann (2016, p. 255).

2 The notion of biomedicalisation, its relation to medicalisation, and its relevance for the project carried out in this book will be further discussed in the epilogue.

3 This closely resembles Parson's (1951) analysis of the sick role. According to Parsons, individuals will only be recognised as sick when they actively seek treatment from medical institutions, and in turn are strongly encouraged to make sense of their suffering only in medical terms. Illich adds to this analysis by stating that this creates a feedback loop through which people become increasingly dependent on medical institutions, because they can no longer make sense of suffering outside of the vocabulary of a medical regime.

4 In fact, also Lupton's (1995, p. 4) distinction between cultural-symbolic norms and medical norms appears to be problematic in light of Foucault's work.

5 The accuracy of Foucault's historical claims has been subject to debate. I will not engage in such debates in this chapter, since my interest in Foucault is sparked by the perspective that he offers on the interrelation of medical and social norms and the conception of the body that underlies this perspective. Therefore, it is not central to my project to determine if Foucault dates certain developments exactly correct and if the processes that he describes are indeed as widespread as he suggests. The debates between Gordon and Erik Midelfort are an interesting entry point to debates about the historical accuracy of Foucault's work, as well as his historiography (e.g., Gordon, 1990; Midelfort, 1990).

6 Like many writers in the 1970s, Foucault was additionally concerned with genetic manipulation and the risks that medicine and the life sciences could pose on a species level or even on the level of life itself. Since my main concern in this chapter is to position Foucault vis-à-vis Illich, I will not discuss these crucial risks. For a discussion of these risks and their relationship to medicalisation, see for instance: Rose (2007b).

References

Canguilhem, G. (1991). *The normal and the pathological* (C.R. Fawcett, trans.). Zone Books.

Carel, H. (2016). *Phenomenology of illness*. Oxford University Press.

Clarke, A.E., & Shim, J.K. (2011). Medicalization and biomedicalization revisited: Technoscience and transformations of health, illness and American medicine. In B.A. Pescosolido, J.K. Martin, J.D. McLeod, & A. Rogers (Eds.), *Handbook of the sociology of health, illness, and healing* (pp. 173–200). Springer.

Conrad, P. (2007). *The medicalization of society: On the transformation of human conditions into treatable disorders*. The John Hopkins University Press.

Erik Midelfort H.C. (1990). Comment on Colin Gordon. *History of the Human Sciences*, *3*(1), 41–45. https://doi.org/10.1177/095269519000300106

Foucault, M. (1978). *The history of sexuality: Volume 1: An introduction* (R. Hurley, trans.). Pantheon Books.

Foucault, M. (1980). Body/Power. In C. Gordon (Ed.), *Power/Knowledge: Selected Interviews and other writings 1972–1977* (pp. 55–62). Pantheon Books.

Foucault, M. (1986). *The history of sexuality: Volume 3: The care of the self* (R. Hurley, trans.). Pantheon Books.

Foucault, M. (2003). *The birth of the clinic: An archaeology of medical perception* (A.M. Sheridan, trans.). Taylor & Francis.

Foucault, M. (2004). The crisis of medicine or the crisis of antimedicine. *Foucault Studies*, *1*, 5–19. https://doi.org/10.22439/fs.v0i1.562

Foucault, M. (2014). The politics of health in the eighteenth century. *Foucault Studies*, *18*, 113–127. https://doi.org/10.22439/fs.v0i18.4654

Gordon, C. (1990). *Histoire de la folie*: An unknown book by Michel Foucault. *History of the Human Sciences*, *3*(1), 3–26. https://doi.org/10.1177/095269519000300102

Hofmann, B. (2016). Medicalization and overdiagnosis: Different but alike. *Medicine, Health Care and Philosophy*, *19*(2), 253–264. https://doi.org/10.1007/s11019-016-9693-6

Homer. (1919). *The Odyssey* (A.T. Murray, trans.). Harvard University Press. (Original work published ca 800 B.C.E.)

Illich, I. (1976). *Medical nemesis: The expropriation of health*. Pantheon.

Illich, I. (2003). Medical nemesis. *Journal of Epidemiology and Community Health*, *57*(12), 919–922. https://doi.org/10.1136/jech.57.12.919

Kusters, W. (2023). On understanding madness: A paradoxical view. *Philosophical Psychology*, *36*(8), 1521–1542. https://doi.org/10.1080/09515089.2022.2146491

Leder, D. (1990). Illness and exile: Sophocles' Philoctetes. *Literature and Medicine*, *9*, 1–11. https://doi.org/10.1353/lm.2011.0157

Lupton, D. (1995). *The imperative of health: Public health and the regulated body*. SAGE.

Metzl, J.M. (2010). Why "against health"?. In J.M. Metzl & A. Kirkland (Eds.), *Against health: How health became the new morality* (pp. 1–13). New York University Press.

Parsons, T. (1951). *The social system*. Collier-Macmillan.

Rose, N. (2007a). Beyond medicalization. *The Lancet*, *369*(9562), 700–702. https://doi.org/s0140-6736(07)60319-5

Rose, N. (2007b). *The politics of life itself: Biomedicine, power, and subjectivity in the twenty-first century*. Princeton University Press.

Svenaeus, F. (2001). *The hermeneutics of medicine and the phenomenology of health: Steps towards a philosophy of medical practice*. Springer.

Toombs, S.K. (1992). *The meaning of illness: A phenomenological account of the different perspectives of physician and patient*. Springer

Wardrope, A. (2015). Medicalization and epistemic injustice. *Medicine, Health Care and Philosophy*, *18*(3), 341–352. https://doi.org/10.1007/s11019-014-9608-3

3 Health, Medicine and Power

Introduction

There is no escape from a medicalised society, which makes it impossible to try to find ways of relating to medicine that are completely extraneous to the medical domain and the power that it exercises. This is how we can summarise Foucault's response to Illich's critique of medicalisation. A *prima facie* reading of this claim suggests that it must be conceded that the experience of healthy embodiment is to a large extent, if not completely, determined by external forces. However, and this will be very familiar to every reader who is slightly familiar with Foucault's work, Foucault's notion of power suggests something different.

The goal of this chapter is to show, via a discussion of Foucault's work on power relations, that to exercise power over something does not equate having complete control over it. In fact, as we will see, Foucault argues against any conception of power that grounds it in one particular object, subject or location from which other objects and subjects are manipulated or dominated. On the contrary, Foucault suggests, "power has its principle not so much in a person as in a certain concerted distribution of bodies, surfaces, lights, gazes; in an arrangement whose internal mechanisms produce the relation in which individuals are caught up" (Foucault, 1977a, p. 202). The question then becomes how the individual is still capable of shaping those relations and/or positioning itself towards them.

Let me be clear here: the aim of this chapter is not to propose a novel reading of Foucault's analysis of power. My goal is instead to mobilise Foucault's work on power to address the specific issue of the extent to which the objectifying power of governmental control determines the experience of healthy embodiment. This was a question Foucault himself was concerned with throughout his career, starting with his earlier works such as *The Birth of the Clinic* and lasted until his later work on biopolitics and technologies of the self. As we will see, addressing this particular question further complicates how to understand the power exercised in the context of public health and biomedicine. This is because any experience of health

DOI: 10.4324/9781003602385-4

presupposes a relationship with one's body, which as we saw in Chapter 1, evades to be controlled completely by the person whose body it is. That is, addressing the question of the extent to which biomedicine and public health can exercise power onto bodies of individuals inevitably entails to also address how the relationship between *Leib* and *Körper* is formed. In the previous chapter, I have suggested that this relationship is mediated by the population(s) that our bodies are made part of. In this chapter, I further outline how this aspects of one's body is subject to power relations.

The chapter is structured as follows. First, I introduce a reading of Foucault in which biomedicine is understood as producing *docile bodies* that are disciplined to behave in a certain manner. Second, I suggest that while the production of docile bodies forms an important part of the experience of healthy embodiment, the experience cannot be reduced to it: the experience of health is not similar to the coincidence with certain disciplinary norms. A discussion of Foucault's notion of governmentality will further explicate how power also gives rise to particular ways of problematisation resulting in desired practices of self-governance. I show how two different ways of self-governance can emerge in response to governmental power: *counter-conduct* and *technologies of the self*. These notions help articulate how the bodies produced within power relations are themselves productive too and can resist and shape the governmental structures in which they are immersed.

§3.1 The Body as Object of Discipline and Surveillance

The idea that bodies of individuals are to be understood in terms of the population that they are part of can be most intuitively linked to Foucault's work on surveillance in *Discipline and Punish*. For instance, Armstrong's (1992) reading of Foucault stresses that since the 18th century, medicine started deploying new techniques to treat illnesses premised on a particular conception of the body, which Foucault terms the *docile body*. This conception of the body underlies the human body as it appears in medicine, particularly in anatomical atlases, and is the condition of possibility for the appearance of the body as a disembodied object in clinical practice in which certain mechanisms leading to disease can be identified.

Following Foucault, Armstrong maintains that the presence of the body as a disembodied clinical object is grounded in the discovery of the body as an object and target of power (Armstrong, 1992, p. 4; Foucault, 1977a, p. 136). This discovery is not to be located in medicine itself but requires to take into account how the body is made present in a wider socio-cultural context. Understanding how the body becomes present as a clinical object hence necessitates to investigate what kind of power is at play here, and how it is being exercised and in what sense it can be described as being docile.

The key term for understanding Foucault's conception of power that underlies the constitution of docile bodies is that of *discipline*. He ties this particular mode of power to the emergence of the Enlightenment, "which discovered the liberties, [but] also invented the disciplines" (Foucault, 1977a, p. 222). The Enlightenment, so Foucault maintains, is marked by two simultaneous and interrelated discoveries. On the one hand, by what he calls the anatomico-metaphysical register which he links to Descartes and that marks the discovery of the body as an object that, just like other objects, is governed by mechanical laws. On the other hand, the Enlightenment is characterised by the discovery of a technico-political register intending to set up regulations by means of calculated methods to control and correct the body's operations (Foucault, 1977a, p. 136).

These latter methods of the technico-political register are what Foucault terms disciplines: those methods that "made possible the meticulous control of the operations of the body, which assured the constant subjection of its forces and imposed upon them a relation of docility-utility" (Foucault, 1977a, p. 137), and are directed "at the formation of a relation that in the mechanisms itself makes [the body] more obedient as it becomes more useful, and conversely" (Foucault, 1977a, p. 138). The connection between the anatomico-metaphysical register and the technico-political register also explains why Foucault characterises discipline in terms of a *micro-physics*: on a macro level, the Enlightenment discovers that all bodies are governed by mechanical laws that make their movement potentially predictable and controllable. The technico-political register is an attempt to cash out this insight on a micro-level—hence the micro-physics—through the development of arrangements and procedures that make individual bodies useful and obedient by means of an installed predictability. Using the term "force" metaphorically, we can say that discipline "increases the forces of the body (in economic terms of utility) and diminishes these same forces (in political terms of obedience)" (Foucault, 1977a, p. 138).

Roughly put, Foucault identifies four general techniques to generate docile bodies (cf. Foucault, 1977a, pp. 141–169): (1) the art of distributions, (2) the control of activity, (3) the organisation of geneses and (4) the composition of forces. In tandem, these techniques discipline by enclosing people in confined spaces with separate sections, each corresponding to different functionalities that are in principle interchangeable: (1) in such spaces, activities are controlled with reference to specific time scales, during which individuals need to perform certain gestures to retain a certain level of productivity that can only be maintained by having a very specific relation to the object of manipulation, (2) the work in these confined, controlled spaces is such that one can constantly improve oneself within the parameters set but is dependent on others in doing so; i.e., one can take steps on a virtually infinite ladder but only by strictly adhering to disciplinary parameters (3) lastly (4), the techniques do not primarily target the individual body, but—and here Foucault borrows from Marx—attempt to "construct a machine whose effect will be maximized by the concerted articulation of the elementary parts of which it is composed" (Foucault, 1977a, p. 164).

The successful execution of these different techniques presupposes an all-encompassing visibility: Foucault's famous panoptical gaze for which Jeremy Bentham's prison design stands as a model. Setting up a model for how to conduct is one side of the coin of discipline, but to ensure that this model is acted upon requires the existence of what Foucault terms a "microscope of conduct" (Foucault, 1977a, p. 173). Bentham's 18th-century design of a panoptical prison functions as an example of such a microscope. The metaphor of the microscope is interesting since having a microscopic view onto something implies to view *selectively*: by means of a microscope, we can only look at an aspect of a particular object but never have a general overview. The key question for the technique of discipline is how to obtain a view of conduct that is both all-encompassing and microscopic. The panoptical model offers an answer to this specific question.

Bentham's panopticon is the opposite of the model of the dungeon; previously, offenders were thrown into a dungeon, thereby rendering them invisible to society and make them suffer in isolation. The panopticon makes a contrary manoeuvre and places prisoners centre stage, thereby making them "perfectly individualized and constantly visible" (Foucault, 1977a, p. 200). In rudimentary form, the design consists of a peripheric building that is divided into cells and a watchtower with wide windows from which all cells are visible. Each cell has two windows, one corresponding to the windows of the watchtower and one at the back of each cell that enables light to travel through each cell. In this way, each cell—and the person imprisoned in it—is visible from the watchtower, and since the light of the watchtower passes through each cell, inmates are continuously aware that they are visible from the watchtower—at least potentially, such that the feeling of being visible is not dependent on the actual presence of someone in the watchtower.

Now, the key for Foucault is that the model of the panopticon is not limited to the prison alone, but "is in fact a figure of political technology that may and must be detached from any specific use" (Foucault, 1977a, p. 205). In the literature of surveillance studies, there is debate about whether Foucault's panoptic conception of surveillance is indeed generalisable and still applies today (e.g., Deleuze, 1992; Galič et al., 2017; Murakami Wood, 2007). Galič et al (2017) make a helpful distinction between *panoptic conceptions* of surveillance that understand surveillance as being confined to particular physical places, and *infrastructural conceptions* of surveillance that understand it in terms of a network that is digital and not confined to a particular form of materiality. The practical effects of these different modes of surveillance might be vastly different, but they have in common the idea that being a body involves to be an objectified part of a given population.

My rationale for discussing Foucault's work on disciplining in the present context is not to suggest that there is a continuity between the methods and effects of surveillance from the 18th century up to the present but rather that, insofar as Foucault's analysis of disciplining makes sense, our experience of our body and its health status is always ingrained into a particular objectifying logic of surveillance that exercises power and cannot be completely controlled. Put differently, the constitution of the body *as part of a population* necessarily involves the constitution of the body *as an object of surveillance.*

§*3.1.1 Surveillance, Biopower and the Governance of Finitude*

The organisation of hospitals is one of Foucault's go-to examples of disciplining in *Discipline and Punish*. However, the relationship between disciplinary techniques, surveillance and medical practice becomes theoretically clearer by linking the notion of discipline to that of population. The constitution of the body as an object of discipline and surveillance, so Foucault argues, makes it present as a site that can be potentially disciplined and controlled. Such practices of control and disciplining are needed to be able to make sure that a population at large displays certain averages considered as desirable (e.g., long life-span, low rate of diseases). Potential disturbances of such averages need to be prevented, which can be done by controlling and disciplining potential outliers, giving rise to "the development of the modern technologies of power that take life as their objective" (Foucault, 1978, p. 152).

The techniques of discipline and surveillance can be linked to the particular project of medicine that understands the bodies of individuals as part of a population, and which was discussed in the previous chapter. This population, then, is conceived of as a large organism of which individual bodies are a part and that must be prevailed by remaining healthy. Put differently, the bodies of individuals are understood as being part of a larger social body that is an object of governance. Hence, the governance of this social body is an affair in which individual organic bodies are considered to be part of a larger organism that can be managed through governmental disciplinary techniques (e.g., Foucault, 1980, p. 55). Again, Foucault links the emergence of this way of governance to a particular historical period, namely the turn of the 19th century, which marks the birth of the medical gaze.

It is primarily this aspect of Foucault's analysis of the relation between medicine and the state that underlies many medicalisation critiques:

medicalisation and the medical gaze presupposed in it turns many aspects of everyday life into medical ones not for the sake of the individual citizen, but for the sake of the interests of states or other institutional or corporate bodies (e.g., Hancock, 2018). That is, the power exercised by the medical establishment, on such views, runs counter to the health-related interests of individuals. As we saw in the previous chapter and the paragraph above, such a critique does not fare well with a Foucauldian conception of power. However, at the same time, we cannot dismiss the factuality of living in societies in which our health and our experience of it are partly structured by disciplinary practices: "The relation of each individual to his disease and to his death passes through the representatives of power, the registration they make of it, the decisions they take on it" (Foucault, 1977a, pp. 196–197).

To further unravel this relationship between health and discipline, it is worthwhile to return to how, according to Foucault, *finitude* has become integrated into disciplinary practices. In *The Birth of the Clinic*, Foucault suggests that an understanding of finitude in terms of disciplining presupposes a particular constitution of the human body in which finitude is made a visible object. Of course, it has always been clear that human beings are finite creatures and that death poses a limit on life. However, there are various ways in which finitude can be concretely understood and linked to an individual body. For present purposes, the two most important understandings of finitude are (1) a transcendent one in which it is understood in terms of a death that forms the negation of life, and (2) an immanent one that takes finitude to be a visible process that is observable in concrete individuals.

When death is understood as the negation of life it is taken to be something that is radically different from all living bodies, and hence cannot become an observable thing in reality: the limits of life transcend those things that are available for human scrutiny. With the emergence of the anatomico-metaphysical register, another perspective on life's limits, which Foucault sees exemplified by the work of the physician Marie-François-Xavier Bichat, opened up, however: Bichat started to dissect corpses, not to reveal particular features of human anatomy to a general public, but instead to be able to trace the pathologies and path of disease that eventually put a limit on life (Foucault, 2003, pp. 140–141; cf. Tierney, 2006, p. 605). As a result, death is transformed from a transcendent moment that is located outside of life into something that is present in life itself and can be made visible when adopting a particular gaze and with the use of the adequate technical means. Finitude, then, while remaining an existential situation in that it affects every living being, becomes also present as an object that can be observed and potentially manipulated.

As indicated earlier, the emergence of the anatomico-metaphysical register was accompanied by the disciplinary techniques of the techno-political register. The combination of the potential to trace the pathway leading up to the limit of life (i.e., by tracing finitude) in individual bodies and an understanding of individual bodies of part of a social body, finitude also becomes a category that can be meaningfully applied to a larger population. Also this population, then, can be constructed as a body that can be dissected, and that is susceptible to particular patterns of disease, in terms of which its finitude can be understood. However, whereas the course of disease in individual bodies can be—at least according to Bichat—partly determined when dissecting corpses, tracing the course of disease in a social body requires a different method; after all, even when understood as an organism, its material constitution does not allow for being subjected to surgical techniques.

While it is not a central theme in *The Birth of the Clinic*, Foucault already suggests here that the anatomico-metaphysical register in which the human body becomes present as a clinical object in which death can be made visible bears the seed for a more encompassing medical gaze:

> For clinical experience to become possible as a form of knowledge, a reorganization of the hospital field, a new definition of the patient in society, and the establishment of a certain relationship between public assistance and medical experience, between help and knowledge, became necessary; the patient has to be enveloped in a collective, homogeneous space.
>
> (Foucault, 2003, p. 196)

For finitude to become visible in the social body, it is needed to develop standards to which individual bodies can be compared. This is only possible through the emergence—the birth—of the clinic in which different patients can be hospitalised and their disease trajectories can be systematically investigated and aggregated. On this basis, it becomes possible to identify something as a "normal" course of disease. However, this is not enough if death is always lurking around. Additionally, it is needed to develop techniques to identify which physiological trajectories *within life* can be considered "normal", such that the trajectories of different diseases and the trajectory of life become distinguishable. Here we immediately see the connection between the anatomico-metaphysical register and the technico-political register: when finitude starts to be conceived of as a clinical object that is visible in life, also the bodies of individuals—the carriers of finitude as one can say—need to be ordered in a certain way for finitude to become visible in the social body. And, as Foucault's panoptical model suggests, to become visible is to become present as an object that can be made subject to disciplinary techniques. This visibility is at the heart of Foucault's notion of *biopower*: the combination of the two registers brings life into the realm of explicit calculations and transforms the lives of concrete individuals by developing disciplinary practices based on them (Foucault, 1978, p. 143).

It is especially the disciplinary aspect of Foucault's thought that is picked up in studies of medicalisation: health becomes an imperative that takes a very narrow shape but that individuals should nevertheless conform to. However, when only conceiving of the human body as being governed as part of a population, we surpass another aspect of Foucault's thought: the fact that the coming into being of the medical body also constitutes it as a site of governance for the individual whose body it is. As we will see, two ways of "governing finitude" can be distinguished: first, the finitude of the state population consisting of bodies as described above, and second, the finitude of my own individualised body. These two different practices of governance correspond to two different ways of conceiving of the body: (1) the medicalised body as *part of a population* that is of sociopolitical concern and (2) the medicalised body as *part of the human being whose body it is*.

§3.2 Resisting Disciplinary Practice

Exclusively understanding medicalisation as a process applying to one's body as part of a population, or even to reduce individual bodies to bodies that are part of a population, is the result of a rather selective reading of Foucault's work. As Tamar Sharon has put it, such critiques maintain that medicine constitutes a

> disciplined subject who ha[s] internalized hegemonic norms of healthy behavior, emphasiz[ing] the disciplinary above the creative aspect of subject constitution in Foucault's work, [and] does not identify how numerous engagements with genetic technologies actually resist disciplinary narratives in unexpected ways.
>
> (Sharon, 2014, pp. 200–201)

And similarly, Crossley has argued—through a critical discussion of both Foucault and Merleau-Ponty—that the very idea of exercising power or inscribing behaviour "is only possible by virtue of an active body, [and] is only of political significance because the body is our (active) way of being-in-the-world. It is because we exist by means of embodied action that it matters how our bodies are treated and how they perform" (Crossley, 1996, p. 114).

And indeed, we find in Foucault the idea that power is not necessarily a form of repression or deprivation but actually acts as a *productive* force: "We must cease one and for all to describe the effects of power in negative terms: it 'excludes', it 'represses', it 'censors', it 'abstracts', it 'masks', it 'conceals'. In fact, power produces; it produces reality; it produces domains of objects and rituals of truth. The individual and the knowledge that may be gained of him belong to this production" (Foucault, 1977a, p. 194). Foucault uses the conceptual pair of *subjection* and *subjectivation* to describe this productive process. On the one hand, power limits certain possibilities and is therefore a form of subjection, while on the other hand, precisely because power produces *subjects*, it produces something that is a candidate for having a degree of freedom that may give rise to resistance to what it is the product of.

Further elaborating on the interrelation between knowledge and power, Lorenzini proposes to understand the techno-political register as involving a particular form of truth-telling, which can "take the form of a 'subjection' (assujettissement) when the individual is required to tell the truth about himself or herself in order for a certain mechanism of power to govern him or her [...], but it can also take the form of a 'subjectivation' (subjectivation) [...] which refers to the construction of oneself as a subject through a certain set of practices or techniques of the self" (Lorenzini, 2016, pp. 70–71). As such, the disciplines do not only constitute subjects that tell relevant truths that can be integrated into governmental mechanisms, but also constitute subjects that can develop techniques to work on themselves that do not need to completely coincide with truths being expected to be told: "it is not that life has been totally integrated into techniques that govern and administer it; it constantly escapes them" (Foucault, 1978, p. 143).

As we already saw in our discussion of Bentham's panopticon as well as the notion of biopower, there is a close intertwinement between knowledge on the one hand and power on the other: disciplining involves not only to be a subject that is supposed to act in a particular manner but also to reveal relevant aspect of oneself in order for disciplinary techniques to be successful. For instance, the management of vaccination rates within a particular social body crucially relies on the ability and willingness of individuals to reveal aspects of their lives relevant to vaccination. And the success of health promotion activities generally is reliant on the extent to which their target can become visible to healthcare professionals. Put differently, health promotion activities co-constitute a particular kind of subject that engages in relevant bodily activities, believes those to be significant, and is willing to share information about these activities with others.

To use Foucault's rather complicated terminology here, the governance of finitude is accompanied with a specific knowledge regime which "form[s] an apparatus (*dispositif*) of knowledge-power that effectively marks out in reality that which does not exist and legitimately submits it to the division between true and false" (Foucault, 2008, p. 19). That is, with "the moment when that which does not exist is inscribed in reality, and when that which does not exist comes under a legitimate regime of the true and false" (Foucault, 2008, p. 20). Implied here is that to live in a society implies to live in a web of power relations that have a ground in knowledge of the involved actors. By means of this knowledge, the reality of relevant phenomena (e.g., health, illness, madness, sexuality) is constituted; it is by means of these relations that certain illnesses can be said to exist or not. This constitution is not determined once and for all but opens up a domain of knowledge that is reportable by and to different subjects (Hacking, 2007). The legitimacy of these phenomena is relative to the web of power relations of which they are a part. For instance, having dyslexia is dependent on the available knowledge of reading skills, their spread in society and the reports of reading skills by the relevant actors. The existence of dyslexia as a real phenomenon is the result of the knowledge gathered in this particular domain. And, if one can legitimately claim to have dyslexia depends on the particular regime they are a part of. Hence, power is not only constraining in that it limits the subject's development, but is also enabling because it provides opportunities for novel ways of self-understanding and to develop a particular relation to oneself and one's conduct.

§3.2.1 *Governmentality and Problematisation*

To understand why Foucault takes power to be productive, it is helpful to show how his analysis of power relates to the broader notion of governmentality. As suggested by Lorenzini, the anatomic-metaphysical register and the techno-political registers emerging in the 17th century have a common goal: the government of the life of human beings in its multiple and interconnected dimensions (Lorenzini, 2023, p. 26). Foucault introduces this notion to counter a potential objection to his suggestion that power is constitutive of subjectivity. If subjectivity is the result of power and cannot be thought independent of it, wouldn't it be impossible to resist power? After all, if power constitutes subjectivity, it seems that the goals and desires of subjects completely coincide with the processes that have produced them. The notion of governmentality serves to answer this objection and to show in what sense subjects can still position themselves in relation to disciplinary practices by problematising them.

Foucault defines the concept of governance as follows: "Governing people, in the broad meaning of the word, is not a way to force people to do what the governor wants; it is always a versatile equilibrium with complementarity and conflicts between techniques which assure coercion and process through which the self is constructed or modified by himself [*sic*]" (2016, pp. 25–26). Hence, to govern does not only entail to develop certain practices or techniques of disciplining and domination, but also to align those with the practices by means of which the self constructs itself. The notion of subjectivation serves to bridge the gap between these through articulating how the subject's own practices of self-construction cannot be thought independently of the disciplinary practices in which it is immersed.

Governmentality can best be understood in terms of the *problematisation* of particular aspects of life. Problematisation is twofold: on the one hand, states can problematise certain practices and exercising power to install new ones. On the other hand, human beings can again problematise such practices themselves and their relation to the installations of power that they are subjected to. As this distinction already indicates, human beings do not problematise in isolation, but always in relation to that what has a particular influence on them. To understand how and why problematisations occur, then, it is needed "to define the conditions in which human beings 'problematize' what they are, what they do and the world in which they live" (Foucault, 1990, p. 10).

This idea of governing by means of problematisation also enables to provide a more nuanced understanding of disciplinary practices. In an essay on his relation to Nietzsche, Foucault writes the following about how the body is not one thing, but rather it emerges different throughout history by being subjected to different governmental regimes: "The body is broken down by a great many distinct regimes; it is broken down by rhythms of work, rest and holidays; it is poisoned by food or values, through eating habits or moral laws; it constructs resistances" (Foucault, 1977b, p. 153). The very practice of breaking down the body into different components can be considered as a way of problematising specific bodily habits, routines and activities that all influence the body's health and conduct. As a result, things like eating habits, working rhythms and the like can be made visible and brought under a governmental regime (i.e., be integrated in disciplinary practices). This is, then, the condition of possibility for any disciplinary practice: by breaking down the body, different objective components are constituted that can fall within the scope of governance.

However, in this process of problematisation, also a specific subject is produced that experiences the different regimes that make up its life and can form new ways to govern those aspects itself. In doing so, it can also start problematising the disciplinary practices that it is subject to and attain a more explicit relation to its own conduct. In the next two sections, I will distinguish between two different ways in which subjects can position themselves vis-à-vis governmental techniques—not by completely eliminating them from their lives but by establishing a particular relation to them. The first is the possibility of counter-conduct, which is grounded in a *collective* desire to be governed differently. The second is what Foucault calls the technologies of the self: the techniques by means of which individuals govern themselves while remaining immersed in a web of power relations. Both ways of relating to governmental practices have in common that their goal is not to evade being governed, but rather to be governed differently, by different means, different techniques and a different kind of leadership.

§3.2.2 *Conduct and Counter-Conduct*

In a lecture given on March 1, 1978, as part of a lecture series at the *Collège de France*, later published in *Security, Territory, Population*, Michel Foucault introduces the conceptual pair of "conduct" and "counter-conduct" to analyse the dynamic of exercising power and resisting it. These interrelated concepts recently gained attention in Foucault scholarship, because of their potential to connect Foucault's earlier work on power to his later work on ethics and subjectivation (e.g., Davidson, 2011). While Foucault introduces these concepts in his analysis of pastoral power throughout the Middle Ages and in the 16th century, they transcend the particular historical domain of (late) medieval Christianity, and remain important to appreciate the exercise of power and the resistance to it up to the present (Foucault, 2007, p. 228; Lorenzini, 2016).

In the March 1 lecture, but also at other places, Foucault links the notion of power to that of conduct and states that the exercise of power in Western society takes the form of imposing a specific form of conduct. He introduces the notion of conduct because it has an internal ambiguity: "Conduct is the activity of conducting (*conduire*), of conduction (*la conduction*) if you like, but is equally the way in which one conducts oneself (*se conduit*), lets oneself be conducted (*est conduit*), and finally, in which one behaves (*se comporter*) as an effect of a form of conduct (*une conduite*) as the action of conducting or of conduction (*conduction*)" (Foucault, 2007, p. 193). As one can see from this definition, conduct has a threefold meaning for Foucault: it entails to conduct someone or something else, to be conducted by someone or something else, but also to conduct oneself. All these three meanings indicate that the activity of conducting (a) is relational at its core and (b) results in a specific kind of behaviour in the person that is being conducted.

Every attempt to govern the conduct of others therefore always implies to stand in a relationship with how a subject wishes to govern himself. This is why, according to Foucault, power is always exercised on subjects that have a certain degree of freedom, and it is precisely because of this that power must be distinguished from violence, coercion or domination. Freedom, here, does not imply the ability to conduct oneself outside of any sphere of power, but instead to be able to engage in a critical self-formation in relation to the forms of conduct that are imposed onto someone. As Foucault puts it, power "is a structure of actions brought to bear upon possible actions; it incites, it induces, it seduces, it makes easier or more difficult; in the extreme it constrains or forbids absolutely; it is nevertheless always a way of acting upon an acting subject or acting subjects by virtue of their acting or being capable of action" (Foucault, 1982, p. 789). Hence, "every power relationship implies, at least *in potentia*, a strategy of struggle, in which the two forces are not superimposed, do not lose their specific nature, or do not finally become confused" (Foucault, 1982, p. 794).

Foucault gives several examples of counter-conduct. One form of counter-conduct that Foucault identifies is the *asceticism* found in monasteries. Through ascetic practices, individuals exercise a strict regime on themselves through which they attempt to obtain full mastery over themselves, their bodies and their sufferings. The goal of such endeavours is to become indifferent to worldly and bodily temptations and to cultivate the ability to constantly master those. Although asceticism is firmly embedded within Christianity, it evades pastoral power because it ultimately consists in the exercise of self on self (Foucault, 2007, p. 205). As a result, there is no external power to which one needs to obey for becoming successful in mastering one's temptations. This placing oneself under a different regime can thus be considered a particular way of conducting oneself against—and this is what makes it *counter*-conduct—the activity of conducting exercised by the church.

A second form of counter-conduct, which can be differentiated from the largely individualising exercise of asceticism, is the formation of *communities*. These communities originate from the rejection of particular aspects of pastoral power and the development of novel practices to replace those. For example, certain communities challenged the pastor's privilege to power and authority on the basis of a definitive and inerasable sign and replaced it with the idea that a pastor's power cannot be independent of his moral character and worldly conduct (Foucault, 2007, p. 208). So, the point of such communities is not so much to remove the pastor from view, but instead to install different pastors that are better suited. Such communities thus remain firmly embedded *within* Christianity, but attempted to work towards a different religious practice to be exercised as a collective. Here, we see that these communities originate from the desire of being conducted differently, by a different form of conduction. In contrast with the practice of asceticism, this form of conducting does not take the shape of a relationship between self and self, but instead as a relationship between self and another type of pastor.

These two examples show that underlying counter-conduct lies the desire to be conducted differently leading to different behaviours. This desire can manifest both through the attempt to develop a particular relationship with oneself, in which another form of conduct arises, but also through the development of a collective that embodies another form of conduction and through which a relation with another forming power becomes possible. This is why Foucault insists that counter-conduct does not imply the negation of power per se and is not grounded in the desire to be not conducted at all and to live in a complete freedom of possibilities. Rather, what unites the activity of counter-conduct is that the "objective is a different form of conduct, that is to say: wanting to be conducted differently, by other leaders (conducteurs) and other shepherds, towards other objectives and forms of salvation, and through other procedures and methods" (Foucault, 2007, pp. 194–195).

A second characteristic of counter-conduct that is clarified through the above examples is that it remains to stand in a relationship with the power(s) that it intends to resist:

> [T]he struggle [against pastoral power] was not conducted in the form of absolute exteriority, but rather in form of the permanent use of tactical elements that are pertinent in the anti-pastoral struggle, insofar as they fall within, in a marginal way, the general horizon of Christianity.
> (Foucault, 2007, p. 215)

The examples of asceticism or the building of novel religious communities still remain to be part of the institute of the church that exercises power on subjects, and the new forms of conducted desired by subjects can, according to Foucault, only be imagined in virtue of the existence of the conduct prescribed by the pastoral regime.

These examples indicate that power is productive of a particular kind of subject that can engage in collective activities of resistance in terms of the things problematised by an existing disciplinary regime. And although the things problematised in contemporary societies are quite different from those at stake in the age of pastoral power, the structure of conduct and counter-conduct remains similar: resistance—as counter-conduct—presupposes an existing form of governance that one not necessarily needs to embrace but which needs to have a presence that is concretely experienced and to which one must consent. And in this moment of consenting to a mode of governance also lies the possibility to desire for different ways of being conducted and to develop new collectives that introduce new norms around which governance is centred.

§3.2.3 *Technologies of the Self*

The governance of bodies not only is an affair of the state that exercises power on its citizens that can be only resisted by means of collective organisation, but also can be considered as a technique of the self that relates to itself. Especially in his later works, Foucault develops this latter theme to articulate that the subject is not entirely subjected and disciplined by external powers, but also actively constitutes itself in relation to both these external powers and itself. He considers this articulation a continuation of ascetic practices in ancient Greece, where "[n]ot to be a slave (of another city, of the people around you, *of those governing you, of your own passions*) was an absolutely fundamental theme" (Foucault, 1997a, p. 285, my emphasis). This brings to the fore an additional theme in Foucault's analysis; not only does governmentality entail not to be subjected to external powers, it also entails not to be subjected to your own passions and desires. In order to avoid both forms of subjection, he holds, the subject needs to develop techniques of the self—or engage in practices of the self—that can be seen as a form of governmentality. This already points to a difference between a perspective that understands the body as an object of (state or market) surveillance and the body as a site of governmentality.

For Foucault, the term "technologies" in "technologies of the self" does not necessarily refer to the material artefacts that people employ to reach certain goals in the external world, but refers to those activities that give an implicit answer to the very basic questions of "What should one do with oneself? What work should be carried out on the self?" (Foucault, 1997c, p. 87).[1] Answering this question, so Foucault maintains, requires to engage in activities of self-governance that enable someone to move in a particular direction while remaining part of a field of contingent forces. This "moving in a particular direction" by attempting to achieve a certain stability, by having the ability to follow a particular alternative within a potential manifold of possibilities, can be considered as subjectivation.

Employing and developing particular technologies of the self is not something that is the result of a pure autonomy that enables to give direction independent of any constraints, but always implies to situate and respond to an already existing field of powers within which someone finds itself. In Foucault's words, technologies of the self "permit individuals to effect by their own means, *or with the help of others*, a certain number of operations on their own bodies and souls, thoughts, conduct and way of being, so as to transform themselves to attain a certain state of happiness, purity, wisdom, perfection, or immortality" (Foucault, 1997b, p. 225, my emphasis). From this definition, three elements stand out: technologies of the self (1) are effects of individuals on their own selves, which (2) transform the self's current state and (3) imply movement towards a certain (desired) goal (the transformation has a direction). Furthermore, this definition also indicates that there is no—or at least that there does not need to be—a clear-cut distinction between practices of counter-conduct and technologies of the self. Both are grounded in the desire for an alternative mode of governance and contribute to the realisation of this alternative.

Whereas Foucault identifies a variety of ways in which work can be carried out on oneself throughout history, all of these have in common that they point to the subject's capacity to resist being a passive target of power relations, and emphasise the potential of the subject to actively steer its own development. Second, subjectivation implies cultivating an ethos that enables one to both identify certain powers that stand in the way of a desired transformation and the ability to position oneself in relation to those powers. Third, subjectivation is described in terms of a struggle without guaranteed success: bodily desires and other forces are always lurking in the background and potentially stand in the way of transforming oneself into a particular direction.

For a subject to be able to engage in such a relationship to oneself and others is not something that one can take for granted, but requires to take care of oneself in a particular way. In his analysis of Foucault's work on subjectivation, Heller notes that Foucault insists that "a subject's ability to speak is ontologically bounded by the discourses through which his or her subjectivity is constructed—a process that is always determined by the subject's location within the specific institutional topography of a particular social formation" (Heller, 1996, p. 91). Because of this, technologies of the self are no spontaneous eruptions of desire but always linked to the presence of existing institutional regimes that have normative impact in that they prescribe what is "normal" conduct. Whereas disciplinary practices are developed to make subjects act in accordance with such prescriptions, the technologies of the self are the result of the desire to take other norms and prescriptions as a starting point for taking care of oneself.

At the same time, Foucault notes, it is both from an analytic and from an experiential perspective rather difficult to make a distinction between technologies of the self and spontaneous experiences (Foucault, 1997b, p. 224). Just as disciplinary practices shape a particular kind of embodied subject that experiences itself and the world around it by being conducted, technologies of the self—which are a form of *self*-conduction—constitute an embodied subject for which its own conduct is not always thematised in experience. Foucault explicates this with reference to principles developed in Stoicism, which he takes to be an example of an attempt to not coincide with external norms. Following the Stoic principles, "you must proceed in such a way that these principles tell you in each situation and, as it were, *spontaneously*, how to conduct yourself" (Foucault, 1997a, p. 286, my emphasis).

Generalising this description of self-conduct, we can see that it aims to become habitually acquainted with the norms and principles one intends to follow, such that they *pre-reflectively* structure one's way of being-in-the-world. Put differently, technologies of the self—just as disciplinary technologies for that matter—are the condition for the pre-reflective structure that can be experienced as a spontaneous reaction to one's environment.[2] And it is precisely for this reason that Foucault's analysis of power becomes relevant for understanding the experience of healthy embodiment and why Foucault's thought is relevant for the phenomenology of health.

§3.3 Conclusion: The Experience of Healthy Embodiment Results from Objectification and Subject Constitution

Let us now return to the issue posed at the beginning of this chapter: to what extent is the experience of healthy embodiment constituted by (institutional) forces outside of the subject's control? Answering this question first requires to acknowledge that the distinction between *Leib* and *Körper* already points to the fact that the objectivity of the body always is a force that cannot be mastered by the experiencing subject, but which has a significant if not crucial impact on one's embodied experience. And since this force can never be fully mastered, one's own body is always partly external to oneself. The present chapter was concerned with the extent to which, given that (pace Illich) there are no extramedical norms that people can orient to, institutional and biomedical norms around health are determining the experience of healthy embodiment.

A key starting point for critiques of medicalisation is the idea that biomedicine and the public health institutions derived from it exercise power on individuals, explicitly or implicitly disciplining individuals in particular ways, and that this exercise of power is not necessarily to the benefit of individuals because it infringes individual freedom. On such accounts, medicalisation is best understood as a means of producing docile bodies by means of disciplinary practices. However, through a detailed reading of Foucault's notion of power, we found that the need to develop disciplinary practices presupposes the existence of a body that is not an object, nor is completely docile, but that has a degree of freedom and has the potential to resist the forces that it is subjected to. This does not imply that it is possible to step out of the context of medicalisation but instead that it gives rise to two different practices of governance in which a different relationship with one's body can be constituted: (1) a relation to the medicalised body as *part of a population* that is of sociopolitical concern and which revolves around disciplinary practices and (2) a relation to *one's own* medicalised body which revolves around counter-conduct and the technologies of the self.

Because of these different relations, there is also the possibility for individuals to participate in practices of governmentality that need not coincide with disciplinary practices but find their ground in the problematisation of those. This points to the possibility of conflict between different practices of governmentality, such that new types of problematisation might occur such that different ways of problematisation start responding to one another. For example, states and markets might develop more "hidden" medicalisation practices by problematising certain aspects of the "social body", which might induce new problematisations by the body of the subject that is disciplined by these practices. As a consequence, the problematisation of medical discourse no longer starts from the position in which a subject approaches a doctor to be healed, but instead from a society that views the subject already in heavily biomedical terms. Because of this, it seems that the difference between the body as part of a population and the body of the human being whose body it is becomes increasingly smaller.

The increase in public health measures from the 19th century onwards contributed further to this process as the destructive potential that are always latently present in every individual body was "expanded in public health discourse to the concept of the social body, the health of which must be protected by its individual members acting responsibly to keep out disease" (Lupton, 1995, p. 75). As a result, "health became a duty, a goal after which people should strive rather than a private, inherent possession of individuals". (Lupton, 1995, p. 38). The means utilised to strive for that goal are—as we saw—to a large extent formulated by the way health is problematised by institutional forms of governmentality. But this is not the end of the story; we can also consider medicalisation as shaping the conditions under which the subject can problematise aspects of its own life, for example, by refusing to submit to hegemonic health norms, or to problematise its own medical body in light of its own finitude. As a consequence, medicalisation can never be considered as a way of governing exercised by the state or market *alone*; it also always potentially involves the governing of oneself by giving rise to new forms of problematisation.

In line with Foucault, we can understand this development of public health in terms of the production of a specific kind of subjectivity. Phenomenologically, the subjectivity is always to be understood as an *embodied subjectivity*. The combination of a phenomenological and Foucauldian analysis shows that one's relation to oneself is doubly mediated by forces it cannot completely master: on the one hand, it involves a relation with one's *Körper* that manifests as an objectivity that intrudes into the experience of healthy embodiment. On the other hand, it involves a relation with one's body as part of a population that similarly manifests as an objectivity that becomes integrated into one's embodied being-in-the-world. And to complicate things further, one's *Körper* and one's body as part of a population stand in a mutually constitutive relation and never appear completely independent of one another. The experience of healthy embodiment, then, does not manifest in terms of a transparent body that needs to be absent from experience but instead in the relations between the different aspects constituting embodiment.

Now that we have sketched a general and abstract account of what healthy embodiment consists in, the next step is to further investigate how contemporary developments in public health and biomedicine shape the experience of health. This will be the goal of the next two chapters that each deal with different, yet interrelated, developments: Chapter 4 discusses how technologies can become part of embodiment and critically positions itself against accounts of technological embodiment that take transparency to be a condition for healthy technological embodiment. Chapter 5 is concerned with the call for a personalised medicine and critically reflects on how personalised medicine introduces certain norms that are integrated into one's experience of healthy embodiment, as well as how this movement envisions the relations between the different aspects of one's body.

Notes

1 In the philosophy of technology, this notion has been interpreted slightly different. It is typically taken to be a response to the material technological artefacts that mediate human subjectivity and the potential of the human subject to position itself in relation to those (e.g., Verbeek, 2011).

2 In this sense, disciplinary practices and technologies of the self are not far removed from what Mauss (1973 [1934]) has called *techniques of the body*: the ways we experience and move our bodies that result from the educational regimes that we were made subject to. For instance, Mauss argues that different styles and experiences of swimming are not explicitly thematised by the swimming person, but do result from particular teaching practices that are forced upon them or that they have chosen to engage in.

References

Armstrong, D. (1992). *Political anatomy of the body: Medical knowledge in Britain in the twentieth century*. Cambridge University Press.

Crossley, N. (1996). Body-subject/Body-power: Agency, inscription and control in Foucault and Merleau-Ponty. *Body & Society*, 2(2), 99–116. https://doi.org/10.1177/1357034X96002002006

Davidson, A. I. (2011). In praise of counter-conduct. *History of the Human Sciences*, 24(4), 25–41. https://doi.org/10.1177/0952695111411625

Deleuze, G. (1992). Postscript on the societies of control. *October*, 59, 3–7.

Foucault, M. (1977a). *Discipline and punish: The birth of the prison* (A. Sheridan, trans.). Vintage Books.

Foucault, M. (1977b). Nietzsche, genealogy and history. In D. Bouchard (Ed.), *Language, counter-memory, practice* (pp. 139–164). Cornell University Press.

Foucault, M. (1978). *The history of sexuality: Volume 1: An introduction* (R. Hurley, trans.). Pantheon Books.

Foucault, M. (1980). Body/Power. In C. Gordon (Ed.), *Power/Knowledge: Selected Interviews and other writings 1972–1977* (pp. 55–62). Pantheon Books.

Foucault, M. (1982). The subject and power. *Critical Inquiry*, 8(4), 777–795.

Foucault, M. (1990). *The history of sexuality: Volume 2: The use of pleasure* (R. Hurley, trans.). Vintage Books.

Foucault, M. (1997a). The ethics of the concern for self as a practice of freedom. In P. Rabinow (Ed.), *Ethics, subjectivity and truth: Of the essential works of Michel Foucault 1954–1984, vol. 1* (pp. 281–302). The New Press.

Foucault, M. (1997b). Technologies of the self. In P. Rabinow (Ed.), *Ethics, subjectivity and truth: Of the essential works of Michel Foucault 1954–1984, vol. 1* (pp. 223–251). The New Press.

Foucault, M. (1997c). Subjectivity and truth. In P. Rabinow (Ed.), *Ethics, subjectivity and truth: Of the essential works of Michel Foucault 1954–1984, vol. 1* (pp. 87–92). The New Press.

Foucault, M. (2003). *The birth of the clinic: An archaeology of medical perception* (A.M. Sheridan, trans.). Taylor & Francis.

Foucault, M. (2007). *Security, territory, population: Lectures at the Collège de France 1977–1978* (M. Sennelart, ed.; G. Burchell, trans.). Palgrave Macmillan.

Foucault, M. (2008). *The birth of biopolitics: Lectures at the Collège de France 1978–1979* (M. Sennelart, ed.; G. Burchell, trans.). Picador.

Foucault, M. (2016) *About the beginning of the hermeneutics of the self: Lectures at Dartmouth College, 1980* (H.P-. Fruchaud & D. Lorenzini, ed.; G. Burchell, trans.). The University of Chicago Press.

Galič, M., Timan, T., & Koops, B.J-. (2017). Surveillance theories from the panopticon to participation. *Philosophy & Technology*, *30*, 9–37. https://doi.org/10.1007/s13347-016-0219-1

Hacking, I. (2007). Kinds of people: Moving targets. *Proceedings of the British Academy*, *151*, 285–318.

Hancock, B.H. (2018). Michel Foucault and the problematics of power: Theorizing DTCA and medicalized subjectivity. *The Journal of Medicine and Philosophy*, *43*(4), 439–468. https://doi.org/10.1093/jmp/jhy010

Heller, K. J. (1996). Power, subjectification and resistance in Foucault. *SubStance*, *25*(1), 78–110. https://doi.org/10.2307/3685230

Lorenzini, D. (2016). Foucault, regimes of truth and the making of the subject. In L. Cremonesi, O. Irrera, D. Lorenzini, & M. Tazzioli (Eds.), *Foucault and the making of subjects* (pp. 63–76). Rowman & Littlefield.

Lorenzini, D. (2023) Foucault, governmentality and the techniques of the self. In M. Tazzioli & W. Walters (Eds.), *Handbook of governmentality* (pp. 22–37). Edward Elgar.

Lupton, D. (1995). *The imperative of health: Public health and the regulated body*. SAGE.

Mauss, M. (1973 [1936]). Techniques of the body. *Economy & Society*, 2(1), 70–88.

Murakami Wood, D. (2007). Beyond the panopticon? Foucault and surveillance studies. In J. Crampton & S. Elden (Eds.), *Space, knowledge and power: Foucault and geography* (pp. 245–263). Ashgate.

Sharon, T. (2014). *Human nature in an age of biotechnology: The case for mediated posthumanism*. Springer.

Tierney, T.F. (2006). Suicidal thoughts: Hobbes, Foucault and the right to die. *Philosophy & Social Criticism*, *32*(5), 601–638. https://doi.org/10.1177/0191453706064899

Verbeek, P.P-. (2011). *Moralizing technology: Understanding and designing the morality of things*. University of Chicago Press.

4 Technological Incorporation and the Experience of Health

Introduction

Power revolves around problematisation. When power is exercised onto a human body with the goal of realising a health goal of some kind, individuals are not simply forced to move in a certain direction. Rather, the individual can organise itself—individually or collectively through counter-conduct against the very forces being exercised upon it. This is why an individual body never completely coincides with the body as part of a population. As we saw in the previous chapter, problematisation does not consist in the negation of power but in positioning oneself against the practices by means of which one is being governed. This is because, following Foucault, governance always involves being subjected to a regime of governance, as well as developing practices of self-governance. Problematisation, then, consists in the relationship between the desired mode of self-governance and the regime that falls partly outside of one's control, be it one's own body's objectivity or the population one is part of.

Moreover, and this is the key topic of this chapter and the following chapter, the governance of health critically involves the use of medical technologies, technological imaginaries and all kinds of potential fusions between bodies and technologies. These technologies constitute a very particular way of problematising health, namely as something that should be governed by means of specific medical technologies. In this chapter, I thematise how technologies shape the constitution of one's body and how bodies are always bodies of biological organisms that, in one way or another, have to adapt to the environment (often by technological means).

The central question to be addressed in this chapter is how the incorporation of technologies into one's body shapes one's experience of health. In elaborating on this question, I challenge the idea that technologies become successfully incorporated by virtue of them being or becoming transparent in experience. The experience of health, then, is not characterised by technological transparency but rather by the experience of friction—or non-indifference—in relation to the environment.

DOI: 10.4324/9781003602385-5

The chapter is structured as follows. First, I introduce one of the key metaphors for describing technological incorporation: that of the cyborg. This notion importantly highlights that technologies are not necessarily foreign to embodiment, but also poses limits on how to understand technological incorporation in everyday life. Second, I introduce the notion of technological mediation to show that technologies mediate intentional relations between humans and world and suggest that they, as a result, can never become completely transparent. Third, this will be further clarified by criticising the notion of cyborg intentionality. Finally, I introduce the work of Georges Canguilhem to point to how health can be understood in the human organism's capacity to exercise its biological normativity, a capacity grounded in an experience of non-indifference or friction. Health, then, consists in the experience of being normative, which is mediated by technologies that are incorporated.

§4.1 The Figure of the Cyborg and Its Limits

One of the central metaphors for understanding fusions between humans and technologies since the middle of the 20th century is the figure of the cyborg. The term "cyborg" is short for cybernetic organism, and its appearance can be traced back to Clynes and Kline's paper "Cyborgs in Space" that appeared in the journal *Astronautics* in 1960. Amidst the space race during the Cold War, Clynes and Kline proposed a new area of research that they thought was promising for how astronauts inhabit space (Kline, 2009). Whereas many research at the time was directed at modifying the environment during space voyages (e.g., modifying the environment of spaceships such that astronauts can inhabit them), they proposed investigating the possibilities of changing the biological make-up of human beings so that they could survive in places previously impossible. They propose the term "cyborg" to describe the result of such modification: "The Cyborg deliberately incorporates exogenous components extending the self-regulatory control function of the organism in order to adapt it to new environments" (Clynes & Kline, 1960, p. 27). This incorporation, they maintained, would make astronauts better equipped for space travel as well as liberate them in what would otherwise be a rather cumbersome environment.

> If man in space, in addition to flying his vehicle, must continuously be checking on things and making adjustments merely in order to keep himself alive, he becomes a slave to the machine. The purpose of the Cyborg, as well as how own homeostatic systems, is to provide an organizational system in which such robot-like problems are taken care of automatically and unconsciously, leaving man free to explore, to create, to think, and to feel.
>
> (Clynes and Kline, 1960, p. 27)

The technological modification of the human biological system is presented as a way of freeing prospective astronauts from being concerned with dealing with the hostilities of the environment in order to direct their attention to those things relevant to space travel: freedom of exploration and deliberation.

Whereas the technological modification of the environment in space makes it remain present as an obstacle that constantly demands attention, the modification of the human body renders the environment and the human body in it transparent, such that intentionality can be directed at those things that are relevant to the project of space travel. Mastering the environment, then, is not the result of technological changes into this environment but the result of the creation of a new entity: the cyborg.

§4.1.1 *Donna Haraway's Cyborg*

A text that has crucially shaped many academic debates around cyborgs is Donna Haraway's *Cyborg Manifesto* that was originally published in 1985. She argues that whereas Darwinian evolutionary biology problematised the strict distinction between humans and animals, the 20th-century mergers of humans and technologies enable to challenge other dichotomies, such as those between organism and machine or between the natural and the artificial. Key to her project is the idea that dichotomies serve to legitimate the domination of those that are constituted as "other", such as women or animals. In challenging such dichotomies and the domination they give rise to, the figure of the cyborg bears the potential of political emancipation and societal change and hence is, according to her, directly relevant to the feminist movement as well as to other emancipatory movements.

Haraway famously defines the cyborg as a "cybernetic organism, a hybrid of machine and organism, a creature of social reality as well as a creature of fiction" (Haraway, 2016, p. 5). The cyborg does not refer to specific individuals displaying certain qualities or having certain characteristics. Instead, "the cyborg is our ontology; [and] it gives us our politics" (Haraway, 2016, p. 7). This figure of the cyborg is dissimilar to the one presented in Clynes and Kline (1960) and neither does it resemble the way cyborgs are typically depicted in popular culture. Haraway's cyborg is not a figure that is stronger than average or in which existing human characteristics are amplified such that the environment can be more effectively dominated but instead is a blasphemy that will challenge the status quo.

Haraway can stage the cyborg as a figure of resistance because she believes that "perhaps, ironically, we can learn from our fusions with animals and machines how not to be Man, the embodiment of Western logos" (Haraway, 2016, p. 52). The Western logos and the rigid dualisms it adheres to have brought humanity in a situation in which certain groups dominate and control others who are defined as "other". When those dualisms are questioned, also existing strategies of control can be effectively resisted, and new relationships between different entities can emerge: "cyborg imagery can suggest a way out of the maze of dualisms in which we have explained our bodies and our tools to ourselves" (Haraway, 2016, p. 67). What is at stake, then, is the development of a new form of self-understanding that enables to more effectively problematise the strategies of power and domination exercised onto people; that is, it bears the potential for new forms of subject constitution.

The cyborg is a figure both of risk and of hope. Of risk because the dissolving of initial dualisms also bears the threat of dehumanisation and more effective control by means of what Haraway calls an *informatics of domination*. Because the human being is no longer a stable, distinctive category, it becomes possible to see it as part of a homogeneous system of information in which they can be treated indifferently. In this case, the bodies of individuals are entirely reduced to being bodies as part of a population. Put differently, the loss of the sacral status of the human being also bears the threat of the development of ever more effective strategies of network management. Of hope because Haraway understands the cyborg as an illegitimate offspring of militarism and patriarchal capitalism: the embodiments of Man par excellence. From these parents, the cyborg was born, and it bears the opportunity to find a new way to speak about the entities inhabiting the world. As Haraway puts it: "[t]he cyborg is not subject to Foucault's biopolitics: the cyborg stimulates politics, a much more potent field of operations" (Haraway, 2016, p. 32). When bodies are no longer understood as singular objects but become present as networks of information, they can also less easily be claimed as a site of discipline. The task of the cyborg, then, is to resist a new homogenising language and instead develop "a powerful infidel heteroglossia" (Haraway, 2016, p. 68).

§4.1.2 *Cyborgs: Creatures of Social Reality or Creatures of Fiction?*

One of the most contested aspects of Haraway's analysis—even for those who otherwise sympathise with her larger political project—is how she navigates between understanding the cyborg as a social reality and as a creature of fiction. More particularly, some argue that—by staging the cyborg as part of a myth—Haraway too easily surpasses the lived experiences and legitimate concerns of those people whose lives depend on an intimate merger with technological devices (e.g., Oudshoorn, 2020; Reeve, 2012). The material reality of cyborgs, then, is considered to be way less heroic than Haraway envisions it to be; after all, someone wearing a pacemaker is not primarily a mythical figure to be mobilised for political emancipation but instead an actually living human being whose own concerns should be taken into account.

Before discussing this critique on Haraway in more detail, it is helpful to briefly consider how Katherine Hayles discusses the background of this problematic. She argues that insofar as the cyborg—or posthuman—is derived from Wiener's cybernetic paradigm, it should be understood as a pattern of information that only accidentally materialised in the embodied beings that humans currently are (Hayles, 1999, p. 2). As a result, there are, in principle, no limits to the direction in which information patterns can develop: our current embodiment is revealed to be a contingent material instantiation instead of a necessary characteristic of a fixed entity called the human being. At the same time, the cyborg is an entity that has a discursive function that invites imagining what we could become from within our current embodied materialisation—regardless of its contingency. This is why the cyborg can be reduced neither to an imaginary discourse such that it becomes a matter of science fiction, nor to a mere material technological practice relevant to medical concerns of current humans (e.g., prosthetics) (Hayles, 1999, pp. 115–116). Precisely because the information metaphor for understanding who we are is so pervasive, the cyborg necessitates asking from the perspective of our current embodied subjectivity how we can transcend our current situation. By definition, then, the figure of the cyborg has an uneasy relationship with the lived reality of those who currently rely on their merger with technologies.

Critics maintain that Haraway's "heroic" interpretation of the cyborg as a figure of political resistance is premised on the assumption that human bodies have a radical openness to technological incorporation. That is, Haraway assumes a transparency of technologies in the experiential lives of users and has a romantic view of the result of mergers between humans and technologies (e.g., Coeckelbergh, 2017, p. 180). However, as has been pointed out by many critical health researchers, such philosophical ideas about cyborgs are often overly optimistic about the extent to which technologies can be incorporated into the human body and implicitly follow the marketing logic behind technological developments (e.g., Cromby & Standen, 1999). Taking as a starting point the lives of those who actually rely on those developments, such critics maintain that ideals about cyborgism (Haraway's included) often too easily surpass the materiality of the bodies that are supposed to be "cyborgian" and do not recognise how they are full of able-bodied assumptions or neglect the actual struggles of disabled people[1] (e.g., Reeve, 2012; Shew, 2020). In other words, when navigating between the aspects of social reality and the aspects of fiction, Haraway leans too much towards the latter.

Shew puts this issue as follows: "In urging us to become cyborgs, Haraway forgets that some of us already are: people on ventilators, prosthetised amputees, wheelchair users, diabetics with insulin pumps, etc. For us, our politicised cyborg identity doesn't come from defying conventional binaries; we are forgotten in both binaries (and in between)" (Shew, 2020, p. 613). For her, as for Reeve, Haraway's focus on the new political action made possible by the figure of the cyborg neglects the materiality of the disadvantages experienced by disabled people (Reeve, 2012, p. 96). The boundaries that Haraway identifies and intends to challenge are not only conceptual or metaphysical boundaries, but are experientially present in the everyday life of disabled people. For instance, the experience of dependency on technologies and the help of others is a key part of life but manifests more drastically in the life of disabled people. And the experience of being excluded from certain aspects of societal life due to unfriendly designs or stigmas is additionally key to understanding what it means to live as a cyborg (Reeve, 2012, p. 108). The Modern categories, those that according to Haraway are blurring only in the second half of the 20th century, have never fit the experience of being disabled, which is why living with a disability is politicised from the start. This political struggle might be heroic, but more important is that this struggle is very real and might not primarily consist in the desire to develop a powerful infidel heteroglossia, but rather in an everyday struggle for recognition.

In her book *The Resilient Cyborg*, Oudshoorn points out that people depending on technologies have developed specific forms of resilience to mitigate their experienced vulnerabilities. In her extensive analysis of people living with pacemakers or defibrillators, she points to the fact that these technological incorporations are not quiet but require active engagement from the people carrying them. This activity is needed because of a variety of the lurking potential for technological malfunction, the re-negotiation of the limits of what one is still able to do, the changing relationships with others due to the visible presence of the implant, or the anxieties resulting from technological uncertainties (e.g., Oudshoorn, 2020, p. 305). Incorporating such technologies hence is not to be understood as simply the result of a surgery after which the everyday cyborg lives happily ever after, but instead as a difficult process of familiarisation requiring to be able to cope with the difficulties that heart implants give rise to. Oudshoorn conceptualises this process as one in which one must ongoingly be resilient to the uncertainties of the changing environment, such that living with heart implants becomes an activity requiring a certain expertise with regard to the frictions resulting from the technology in question instead of a passive integration of a transparent technology.

Generally put, the critiques on Haraway discussed above are directed at the idea of technological transparency, leading to three key assumptions underlying the ideal of the cyborg, namely that technologies (1) allow for being incorporated in the human body rather unproblematically, (2) attain a high degree of transparency in virtue of this incorporation and (3) that the health of the cyborg figure is considered to be relative to the degree of technological transparency.

§4.2 Postphenomenology and the Impossibility of Technological Transparency

In the previous section, I have suggested that many interpretations of the cyborg presuppose some form of technological transparency. In this section, I will further explain what this term exactly entails to be able to highlight why it gives rise to problematic assumptions about the relation between humans and technologies. To do so, I turn to the work of Ihde, who is often considered to be the founding father of postphenomenology, which is a prominent school of thought in the philosophy of technology. As the name of the school already suggests, postphenomenology has its roots in phenomenology and its interest of carefully describing human intentionality. However, it departs from phenomenology because, according to postphenomenologists, most 20th centry phenomenologists have the tendency to conceive of science and technology as hegemonic forces suppressing human authenticity and that need to be eliminated from view to come up with descriptions of intentionality.

In contrast with such a view, postphenomenologists maintain that our intentionality is fundamentally shaped by the products of science and technology, such that eliminating those from view implies eliminating one of the crucial aspects of human existence and experience. The notion of technological mediation is key to how postphenomenologists understand the ways in which technologies shape intentionality, as they typically maintain that technologies are best characterised as mediators of human-world relationships. This is a constant characteristic of all technologies, ranging from prehistoric hand axes to current imaging technologies in biomedicine, to smartwatches used to track health-related parameters.

Let us now further unpack the idea of technological mediation. This notion expresses that technologies are not mute tools that enable users to realise pre-set goals more effectively, but instead actively shape how embodied individuals experience and understand themselves and the world around them. Technologies texture the world in which humans are situated, thereby shaping both the subject experiencing the world and the world that is experienced by the subject. This is interpreted as a form of co-constitution in which technologies constitute both subjectivity and objectivity by mediating particular relations between these two poles (de Boer, Kudina, & Hoek, 2018; Verbeek, 2005).

For instance, Functional magnetic resonance imaging (fMRI) scans shape how cognitive psychologists understand cognition, thereby constituting both cognition as a particular kind of object to be interpreted in terms of brain activity, as well as particular kind of subject that observes cognition through this particular lens (de Boer, te Molder, & Verbeek, 2020). Or (maybe) closer to home, word-processing programmes and typewriters each shape differently how one engages with writing a text. Whereas typewriters invite careful writing and think before writing a sentence, a word-processing programme invites a writer to start writing immediately because it is much easier to make corrections. In each case, the relationship between writer and text takes shape differently as a result of the mediating technologies involved (Ihde, 2010, pp. 74–76).

Ihde explains these different mediations with reference to an amplification-reduction structure that is inherent to the intentional relationships that technologies help constituting (Ihde, 1979, p. 21). This structure is already visible when using a simple tool such as a knife to slice bread. The knife mediates one's experience of the bread by amplifying certain features of it (e.g., the hardness of the crust is amplified), while reducing other features (e.g., the temperature of the bread). Similarly, more complex technologies such as microscopes used in a cytology laboratory amplify the particular anomalies present in cell structures and invite cytologists to understand disease in terms of these pathologies, thereby tending to focus less on patients' lived experiences of illness (e.g., Forss, 2012).

While seemingly straightforward, such amplifications and reductions tend to remain invisible precisely because our interactions with technologies can be characterised in terms of ready-to-handness. Postphenomenologists typically follow Heidegger's distinction between the ready-to-hand and the present-at-hand here and maintain that our primary interactions with the world are ones in which the tools we use remain *transparent*.[2] That is, they are already presupposed and embedded into existing systems of habits and signification, and are not thematised in experience. Since we experience the world through technologies, they are typically *transparent* in use such that they do not become a focus of our attention, as we are directed at the world experienced through the technology instead of at the technology itself (e.g., Ihde, 2010, p. 14; Van Den Eede, 2011; Wellner, 2020).

The ways in which technologies, from a postphenomenological point of view, become transparent in use is key for understanding the mergers between humans and technologies. Postphenomenologists tend to follow Merleau-Ponty and maintain that the limits of the body do not coincide with our skin and that tools and technologies can become part of one's body schema and as such shape motor intentionality. As Rosenberger has shown, this transparency is not given but requires training in particular skills that are necessary for successful incorporation, and as a result of which the technology in question disappears from experience (i.e., becomes transparent) (Rosenberger, 2012). And on top of that, as exemplified in Oudshoorn's analysis of pacemakers, incorporation is relative to the material qualities of the body merging with a particular technology, as well as the social context in which the merger takes place. Generally put, transparency is always relative to a particular user and context in which the merger occurs.

And precisely because the use context is always subject to change (and has a specific temporality), the transparency of technologies can never be complete or total; the potential to make them thematic in our experience is always latently present. However, at the same time, it can be noticed that many interpretations of human-technology mergers tend to slip (either explicitly or implicitly) from what Ihde calls the quasi-transparency that is characteristic for how technologies are typically become incorporated into a technofantasy of total transparency (Ihde, 2012, p. 376). He links this to a broader desire of merging completely with technology: a wish for total transparency, which, in Ihde's view, "secretly rejects what technology is and overlooks the transformational effects which are necessarily tied to human-technological relations" (Ihde, 1990, p. 75).

The desire for total transparency would be to have the transformative effects of technology without having the ability to be aware of them or to thematise them, which, in Ihde's view, would be the equivalent of there being no technology at all. After all, it is precisely the transformative effects that result from technological mediations which constitute a novel meaningful relationship with the world. And moreover, since the transparency of technologies is the result of in*corpo*ration, a previous form of embodiment must be assumed: there must exist something in which technologies can be incorporated and for which they can become transparent.

Insofar as narratives around the cyborg, be they those of Haraway or those of techno-optimists maintaining that technological artefacts are the key to solving medical issues, assume complete transparency of technology, they tend to ignore—or at least downplay—what it means for a technology to be incorporated. On the one hand, this ignorance generates unrealistic expectations for what (medical) technologies can and cannot do, while on the other hand, they also surpass how they shape the subjectivity of users and the way the world appears to them as a meaningful whole. Moreover, and this is especially pertinent for Haraway's project, when technologies indeed become completely transparent and the figure of the cyborg becomes "complete", it also seems, since the merger and its effects escape our attention, difficult to think of the cyborg body as a site of resistance, as it is difficult to obtain a critical relation with those technologies that are constitutive of the cyborg. In sum: insofar as technologies can be adequately understood as mediators that are constitutive of both subjectivity and objectivity, embodiment has a certain openness that makes incorporation possible, but this openness can never be completely closed. In the next section, I will further outline how technologies shape embodied intentionality by discussing how we must understand embodiment both in terms of openness and closure.

§4.3 Cyborg Intentionality and Its Limits

To further elaborate on the issue of technological incorporation, this section provides a critical analysis of the idea of *cyborg intentionality*. Cyborg intentionality can be roughly defined as the constitution of a particular human–world relation that is shaped by how technologies are incorporated in the human body. These particular forms of incorporation, then, are taken to disclose the world in a specific way, thereby giving rise to specific technological mediations. In this process, both the (cyborg) subject and the world, as well as how it acts, speaks and understands itself in this world attain a specific "shape".

The notion of cyborg intentionality was put forward by Verbeek (2008) who makes a distinction between technologies that are embodied and those that are incorporated: "Technologies used, like telescopes and hearing aids, help to constitute us as different human beings, whereas technologies incorporated constitute a new, hybrid being—which could, in principle, also use technologies which help to constitute us as different 'transhumans'" (Verbeek, 2008, p. 392). Examples of the technologies of incorporation that Verbeek refers to are microchips that enhance the vision of people who are visually impaired or pharmaceutical drugs that alter one's mood (e.g., antidepressants). According to Verbeek, these technologies are not embodied in the way Ihde understands the term, because they have a different temporality and are not connected to specific contexts of use: microchips are not linked to particular kinds of activities and neither can users easily choose to be "de-coupled" from them. Whereas it is still, at least in principle, possible to distinguish between the human and the technological aspects in the case of embodiment relations, this is no longer possible for our relations with microchips or drugs, in which case "humans and technologies form a new experiencing entity" (Verbeek, 2008, p. 391): it is this entity that can be called a cyborg with a distinctive kind of intentionality.

A distinction can be made between phenomenological and the ontological readings of Verbeek's notion of cyborg intentionality: the notion entails phenomenologically that there are instances in which we can note a distinctive experiential unity in particular mergers of humans and technologies, such that the difference is noted neither from a first-person perspective nor from a third-person perspective. Interpreted ontologically, the implications of the notion are stronger because this interpretation entails that it is in principle no longer possible to distinguish between the human and the technological aspects and that something distinctively new emerges which forms a stable referent for the term "cyborg". Or put differently, phenomenologically speaking cyborg intentionality is circumstantial, whereas ontologically it is lasting.

These different interpretations demand different things from cyborg technologies in terms of their transparency. The phenomenological interpretation commits to the idea that there are instances in which "cyborg" technologies (e.g., pacemakers) are transparent in that they withdraw from experience, such that human and technology form an experiential embodied unity that is a gateway for meaningful interaction with the world. The ontological interpretation is committed to an interpretation of transparency with a different temporality. In this case, technologies need not only to be experientially transparent in particular instances but become integrated into embodiment in such a way that it is no longer possible to distinguish between human and technology and that a novel experiential embodied unity is constituted, which itself forms the basis for other interactions with the environment. To put it in Husserlian terms: the zero-point of orientation itself changes.

§4.3.1 *The Limits of Transparent Embodiment*

When indeed a new entity is created through the merger of humans and cyborg technologies (as the ontological interpretation of cyborg intentionality would have it), the technologies in question are interpreted as totally transparent. But to what extent does this ontological interpretation fall prey to what Ihde identifies as the technofantasy of total transparency? That is, would it be grounded in a misconception of what technologies actually are, thereby overlooking their transformational aspects?

To answer this question, it is helpful to highlight that Ihde's criticism of the desire for total transparency is primarily directed at fantasies about virtual technologies and is written in the context of debates concerning whether virtual reality can supplant or replace real life. Ihde's interventions in such debates typically take our human embodiment as a starting point and ask about the possibility of leaving our embodied being-in-the-world. His argument against the replacement of real life with virtual reality can be summarised as follows: when we imagine doing something that we have not in fact done (say, parachute jumping), we already imagine ourselves as another that we actually are not. This can be done from an embodied and a disembodied mode: the first mode prioritises felt characteristics such as the wind rushing in one's face, the vertigo in one's stomach, whereas the second mode sees an object version of oneself entering an airplane, gaining a certain altitude, etc. And even if the embodied mode of imagination might be more intense or rich in description, it remains contingent on the possibility of adopting a theatrical view onto oneself *from within the lifeworld* in which I am present as an already embodied being. Both virtual reality and its counterpart "real life" "are part of the lifeworld, and VR [virtual reality] is thus both 'real' as a positive presence and a part of RL [real life]" (Ihde, 2002, p. 13).

According to Ihde, any description or imagination of technologically induced virtuality has a similar structure. Also fantasies about our bodies in virtual environments are dependent on the lifeworld, which both enables us to develop certain imaginations and puts constraints on the extent to which such imaginations can be realised. On the one hand, the types of image-objects that we can realise are dependent on the technological developments that spark our imagination. For instance, dreams of mind-uploading are contingent on the material presence of computers and the possibility to store large amount of data. On the other hand, because such imaginations are grounded on both the fragile materiality of a certain technological environment and on an embodied being for which image-objects are constituted (cf. Besmer, 2015). Accordingly, the virtual can never replace real life, just as little theatre can replace actual life: the experiencing subject always remains capable of minimally detecting this distance.

From this argument, Ihde concludes that:

> VR bodies are thin and never attain the thickness of flesh. The fantasy that says we can simultaneously have the powers and capacities of the technologizing medium without its ambiguous limitations, so thoroughly incorporated into ourselves that it becomes living body, is a fantasy of desire.
>
> (Ihde, 2002, p. 15)

The question now becomes if this argument can be extrapolated to the context of the cyborg technologies discussed earlier, and if those actually can "attain the thickness of flesh".

To address this issue, it is instructive to discuss Kirk Besmer's analysis of embodying a cochlear implant. This is a technology developed for people who experience deafness or profound hearing loss. It can give those people auditory sensations by stimulating the auditory nerve directly (Besmer, 2012, p. 302). He argues that it can take years before users of cochlear implants actually get used to the cacophony of sounds they suddenly start experiencing and become able to discriminate sounds within an environment of noise. "Normal" hearers have a passive embodied understanding of their auditory environment, such that discriminating sounds does not require active interpretation. Rehabilitation in terms of hearing would then consist of acquiring this passive understanding by integrating the act of interpretation into one's perceptual scheme.

The transition that might result from this process of integration is, to speak with Besmer, "not merely the addition of new sounds superimposed on a stable, silent world; instead, a new world emerges around a new body. It is a complete re-worlding" (2012, p. 307). This is because the new experiential unity emerging through the cochlear implant is perceptually completely dissimilar to the previous unity. Whereas, for instance, someone using a cane is in principle capable of having tactual sensations, the wearer of the cochlear implant has no auditory sensations at all without it, which is why Besmer speaks about this "complete re-worlding". In this case, so it seems, the "cochlear implant body" does attain "the thickness of the flesh" such that a new way of embodied being-in-the-world is constituted.

In the case described by Besmer, it seems that at least, technologically, there is the possibility of transparency such that the merger between human and technology constitutes a new entity. However, even if the cochlear implant (and the sounds that it constitutes)—contrary to Oudhoorn's descriptions of wearers of pacemakers—becomes part of a passive embodied scheme, this does not necessarily entail that the wearer's body and the world they inhabit are completely transparent. After all, as Merleau-Ponty already noted in the *Phenomenology of Perception*: "What allows us to center our existence is also what prevents us from centering it completely, and the anonymity of our body is inseparably both freedom and servitude" (Merleau-Ponty, 2012, p. 87).

With this realisation, we have circled back to a critical general issue in the phenomenology of embodiment: even if technologies can become completely transparent such that a new constant experiential unity is constituted, this embodied unity itself—as a vehicle enabling meaningful interaction with the world—can itself not be fully understood in terms of its "absent presence" (Leder, 1990). And insofar as the notion of "cyborg intentionality" is parasitic on this particular understanding of "healthy" embodiment, it insufficiently recognises how the human body is constituted. As I have shown in previous chapters, this constitution inevitably involves a relationship between *Körper*, *Leib* and Body as Part of a Population. Of course, these different elements can form an experiential unity at some point in time, but this unity is fragile and subject to constant change. As a result, total transparency remains being a fiction.

§*4.3.2 From Transparency to Friction*

Ihde typically understands embodiment in terms of transparency and holds that the world is constituted in virtue of this transparency. In his work, embodiment often appears as the gateway for meaningful interaction with the environment, such that it replaces the traditional notion of "consciousness" as making possible the encounter with the environment and the objects in it (e.g., Ihde, 2010, p. 65). As I will show in this section, this can be considered a general limitation of the postphenomenological understanding of the human body. For, as we saw in the previous chapters, there is a plethora of cases in which our body refrains from being transparent, and this can happen for different reasons.

We find clues in Ihde's work for how our embodied pre-reflective presence is culturally shaped in his distinction between "body one" and "body two". On the one hand, we can describe embodiment in terms of our motile embodied being-in-the-world; Merleau-Ponty's "I can" (body one). On the other hand, we are also bodies in a social and cultural sense, such that certain aspects of our body have certain significances: in many contemporary societies, the female breast carries sexual significance, whereas this significance is reserved for the ankle in other times and places. For Ihde, "[t]raversing both body one and body two is a third dimension, the dimension of the technological" (Ihde, 2002, p. xi).

While recognising that the existence of a particular experience of one's own body is shaped through cultural expectations and the gaze of others that might problematise transcending *into* the world, he does not explicitly thematise how this experience can be shaped by technological developments (Ihde, 2002, p. 18). This is because he is primarily interested in revealing how technologies open up new capabilities of interacting with the world by being transparently integrated into our embodiment, or on how embodiment puts limits on mergers between humans and technologies. However, what he does not focus on are investigations of how technologies also give rise to particular experiences *of* one's own body that constitute the world in a particular manner. An analysis of the experience of health and illness helps explicate this other way in which human–world relationships are mediated by technologies.

The knife thus cuts two ways: on the one hand, postphenomenology allows for augmenting the phenomenological approach and the medicalisation view by showing that there is no universal pattern to which technologies in medicine conform. On the other hand, however, a better understanding of how one's own body is experienced in health and illness allows for showing that the constitution of "world" crucially involves—besides the relationship between humans and technologies—the relationship with one's own body; a relationship that is in turn *also* mediated by technologies. As a result, just as an analysis of health and illness is incomplete without taking into account the technologies that mediate our experience of it, it does remain so too without analysing the particular constitution of one's own body in the experience of health.

Key for understanding the experience of health—be it in light of technological incorporation, be it in light of the *Leib-Körper* distinction, be it in light of medicalisation and the body as part of a population, is that one never completely coincides with a particular aspect of one's body. As a result, the experience of health does not give rise to complete transparency. Moreover, as is made clear by my discussion of how technologies mediate the human–world relation, the experience of health also crucially involves a relationship with one's environment. In the next section, I will introduce the work of Canguilhem, most notably his notion of biological normativity, to articulate what qualifies as a healthy relationship with the environment. As we will see, this requires leaving the idea of bodily transparency behind and moving to an understanding of health that is characterised by *friction*.

§4.4 Georges Canguilhem: Health as Biological Normativity

The notion of cyborg intentionality and the postphenomenological framework in which it is embedded are premised on a particular understanding of embodiment in which the emphasis is on how bodies (interpreted in terms of *Leib*) function as a vehicle for meaningful interaction with the world. However, the fact that technological embodiment is not always equally successful already indicates that there is also an aspect of the body that resists incorporation. And this bodily resistance is also *embodied* in that it might prevent an individual from understanding or experiencing their body as a vehicle for meaningful interaction with the environment.

The goal of this section is to show how Canguilhem's understanding of health enables to characterise the relationship between *Leib* and *Körper* in terms of the extent to which an individual experiences their relationship with the environment as healthy. Canguilhem wrote extensively on how to understand individuals as healthy or ill beyond the internal, detectable and measurable processes taking place in the human body by focusing on the dynamic relationship between organism and environment.[3] For Canguilhem, the starting point is that, regardless of which technologies are incorporated into human bodies, they are always biological organisms intending to realise key biological values (e.g., food, survival, reproduction). Realising these values requires adapting to and adjust the environment to a certain extent. In this sense, the body can be considered as a technique that allows for the realisation of such values.

In the case of the human organism, the values to be realised might not be as narrow as those suggested in general biological approaches, but might also include things that are explicitly experienced as meaningful. Yet, also in this case, it seems that realising these meaningful things requires adaptation. However, in the very process of incorporating and using technologies to adapt to the environment, organisms simultaneously *adjust* the environment. It is because of this, so I suggest, that the incorporation and use of technologies is not a *passive form* of adaptation, but instead allows *actively* adjusting the environment in which the organism lives. This, in turn, has consequences for what we would take to be the "healthy cyborg" that now can no longer be characterised in terms of degrees of technological transparency, but instead in terms of its capacity to adapt to the environment and adjust the environment in this process.

For Canguilhem, the process of adapting and adjusting to the environment is key to understanding the experience of health. This relationship with the environment is characterised by what he calls a *biological normativity* on the side of the organism. Biological normativity is, according to Canguilhem, grounded in biological life, which is fundamentally characterised by a *non-indifference* to the environment, meaning that they react more or less spontaneously to those aspects of the environment that obstruct their preservation. Organisms do so by imposing new norms on themselves or on the environment, which result in a modification of either the organism's conduct or the environment (Canguilhem, 1991, p. 126; cf. Sholl, 2016). For Canguilhem, the non-indifference of organisms is a basic characteristic of biological life, which, as he says, "is far removed from [...] an indifference to the conditions which are made for it; life is polarity" (Canguilhem, 1991, p. 128). In this sense, life is considered to be a norm-setting activity in constant struggle with that which prevents the realisation of key biological values (e.g., food, survival, harm avoidance) and, hence, is inherently future-oriented (Trnka, 2003).

In line with this idea, health is understood as a particular expression of normativity that structures how an organism relates to its environment and which is constitutive of the extent to which it can adapt to and adjust the environment (Canguilhem, 1991, p. 77). Health constitutes "the possibility of transcending the norm, which defines the momentary normal, the possibility of tolerating infractions of the habitual norm and instituting new norms in new situations" (Canguilhem, 1991, p. 115). These norms are not equivalent to mechanistic functions that stand in a causal relationship with certain environmental mechanisms. Such an understanding of norms mistakenly takes the environment in which organisms live to be a (fixed) *physical* environment; as an already constituted fact. However, biologically speaking, "the organism is not thrown into an environment to which he must submit, but he structures his environment at the same time that he develops his capacities as an organism" (Canguilhem, 1991, p. 284). Hence, the environment to which the individual relates is no theoretical abstraction remaining unchanged over time but is instead relative to the organism's ability to modify it and/or adapt to it. Since organisms continually move through different environments, they are in continuous need to exercise this ability in relation to different environmental circumstances. Health, then, for Canguilhem, is an expression of the organism's capacity to cope with a multiplicity of environments that the organism inevitably faces, each asking for a certain response; it "is a margin of tolerance for the inconstancies of the environment" (Canguilhem, 1991, p. 197).

Biological normativity is a response to the inconstancies of the environment. For Canguilhem, being normative implies exercising norms that enable to experience specific environments as normal. In Foucault, we already encountered the idea that normality or normalisation forms an integral part of the way of the form of governance that is present in scientific medicine and public health. Canguilhem, contrary to Foucault, does not primarily link normalisation to governmental practices but understands it as an integral part of life itself that is experientially present to every living organism. The experience of health is not only the result of the production of a particular subject but manifests in the ways in which an organism expresses itself as a particular individual body that continuously represents, exercises and evaluates its powers and limits in a dynamic environment.

For example, being healthy involves being tolerant to weather changes (or changes in climate when moving to another country) without experiencing those as a threat to the organism's capacity of organisation. Or the organism might employ certain technical means to build houses for shelter, thereby structuring the environment it needs to adapt to. An extreme example of the reverse of the capacity for adaptation would be a foetus only capable of surviving in an incubator, and which is too weak to be exposed to the environment outside of it and passes away in this very exposure. Whereas the foetus can tolerate one specific technological environment, it passes away when it has to leave it. Hence, the way in which organisms adapt to and adjust the environment is fundamentally intertwined with the use of technologies around which specific milieus are constituted. As a result, understanding technics is key to understanding health:

> [W]e cannot clearly understand how the same man with the same organs feels normal or abnormal at different times in environments suited to man unless we understand how organic vitality flourishes in man in the form of technical plasticity and the desire to dominate the environment.
> (Canguilhem, 1991, p. 201).

In health, the organism can execute its powers without actively being constrained by the environment in which it lives. In this case, "life [is] being lived in the silence of the organs", such that the healthy individual is someone "who adapts silently to his task, who lives the truth of his existence in the relative freedom of his choices" (Canguilhem, 2012, p. 49). In illness, an organism experiences a qualitative transformation in its relation to the environment that makes it feel "inferior to the task which the new situation imposes on him" (Canguilhem, 1991, p. 182). The sick organism experiences a qualitative transformation when feeling sick because disease is the becoming present of a new *norm* that leads him or her to differently evaluate the powers and limits when relating to a given environment. In illness, the organism does not cease to be normative but instead institutes a new norm, making that it feels unfit to "tolerate and compensate for the aggressions of the environment" (Canguilhem, 2012, p. 49). The new norm gives rise to a different evaluation of one's powers and limits, such that a different relationship with the environment emerges that is experienced as intolerable. It is this new norm that forms a criterion for making the distinction between health and illness, because it marks a new way of being non-indifferent to the environment.

§4.4.1 *Self-Regulation and the Difference between Illness and Anomaly*

According to Canguilhem, for the human organism, being healthy implies not only to live life "in the silence of the organs—it is also life lived in the discretion of social relations. If I say [...] that I am unwell, people want to know how and why; they wonder or ask me whether I am registered with social security" (Canguilhem, 2012, pp. 49–50). As a human organism, so Canguilhem suggests, one lives in a particular society in which certain norms are present about what constitutes a "healthy life", and which are influenced by medical developments. In his words: "the body as understood by the people has always been indebted to the body as understood by the faculty of medicine" (Canguilhem, 2012, p. 51).

As we saw in the previous chapter, this "being indebted" importantly consists of medicine exercising certain norms about health: medicine shapes what are taken to be forms of appropriate self-governance. This prompts the question of to what extent social norms, including the ones put forward in preventive medicine (e.g., a certain average lifespan in a given population), play a role in shaping what is experienced as a healthy norm. Answering this question requires considering how Canguilhem distinguishes between the way organisms and societies are organised. In making a distinction between the two, he critically reacts against philosophers and biologists that compare the organisation of society to the organisation of organisms (e.g., the philosopher August Comte, or the physiologist Walter B. Cannon). According to Canguilhem, this comparison is fundamentally mistaken because it fails to distinguish between two different forms of regulation: a self-regulation, and a form of regulation that is external to the existence of something, where the former applies to organisms and the latter to societies.

The origin of organismic regulation is to be found in the organism's non-indifference to the environment that manifests in the organism's activity of norm-setting, which Canguilhem calls, as indicated before, biological normativity. Organisms "live as a whole and [are] not [...] able to live except as a whole. This is made possible by the existence [...] of a set of apparatuses or mechanisms of regulation whose effect consists precisely [...] in the persistence of the organism as a whole" (Canguilhem, 2012, p.

72). Societies, by contrast, lack self-regulation, such that it is needed to collectively and continuously debate in accordance with which ideal a society should be regulated. In the absence of a clear ideal, societies are "always out of order, because [they] are deprived of [a] specific apparatus of self-regulation" (Canguilhem, 2012, p. 77). Societies, then, are always characterised by a certain incompleteness because their functioning is dependent on something external, such that they can never be a completely organised whole. This would make it arbitrary to rely on social valuations as a way of distinguishing health from illness: "To define abnormality in terms of social maladaptation is more or less to accept the idea that the individual must subscribe to the fact of [a given] society" (Canguilhem, 1991, pp. 282–283). This is why Canguilhem does not conceive of "healthy organisation" in terms of a form of individuation that coincides with socially valued ends.

The distinction between societal and organismic organisation has consequences for how the distinction between health and illness can be made. This can be clarified through the distinction between *illness* and *anomaly* made by the Gestalt psychologist Kurt Goldstein, whose work greatly influenced Canguilhem's. Goldstein maintains that whereas concepts like health and illness are norms of living for the concrete individual, the notion of anomaly points to an external observation of an organism that compares it against the species that it belongs to and/or the specific groups (e.g., nationality, age group, neighborhood, level of education) that it is part of (Goldstein, 1995, p. 344). The concept of anomaly thus suggests that it is possible to make a quantitative distinction between the normal and the pathological.

According to Goldstein and Canguilhem, however, such an interpretation fails to notice that health and illness must be considered relative to how organisms regulate themselves and exercise their norm-setting capabilities. Different ways of self-regulating, as we saw, constitute the experience of being fit or unfit to exercise its powers on the environment. It is this qualitative experience that, for Canguilhem, functions as a demarcation criterion between health and illness. While it is perfectly possible that the social norms and valuations shape the experience of illness, they are in themselves neither necessary nor sufficient conditions for demarcating between health and illness. This demarcation takes place on the level of the organism that might or might not experience its relations with the environment as pathological (i.e., as instantiating a qualitative transformation through which it feels unable to tolerate and compensate for the aggressions of the environment).

Medicine should, according to Canguilhem, not be concerned with attempting to make someone who experiences illness return to a presumably normal state relative to the species to which it belongs, nor with ideals derived from societal averages. Rather, maintaining individuality presumes both that the organism is capable of having a certain stability in relation to the variety of environments it faces, and that it does not completely integrate with social norms and averages but is capable of organising itself in relation to those. In both cases, it is key for the organism to maintain a certain degree of individuality that makes norm-setting possible and prevents it from completely merging with one particular environment.

What emerges from Canguilhem's analysis of health and illness is that the environment in which the organism is situated is not necessarily welcoming such that humans can unproblematically transcend into it. Rather, the environment is always to a certain extent hostile, and exercising biological normativity is a way of dealing with this hostility. And since the environment is not one unified homogeneous mass but always subject to change, the human organisms must be able to be normative in a variety of environments that are non-indifferent to them. Technologies, then, change both the environment—or world—that people inhabit and constitute new ways of being non-indifferent. Besmer's analysis of cochlear implants is a good example of this: his description of the changes occurring as a result of those implants in terms of a "complete re-worlding" (Besmer, 2012, p. 307) indicates that incorporating technologies gives rise to new forms of friction that demand people to exercise new norms onto the environment. This friction is mediated by technologies that, even if they are physically transparent, still shift the embodied experience of being-in-the-world and shape the experience of health.

§4.5 Conclusion: Adaptation and Problematisation—Technologies and Changing Milieus

I started this chapter by pointing to the intimate relationship between power and problematisation. The idea that technological incorporation is to be understood in terms of friction can be linked to the idea of problematisation: technologies shape the way(s) in which humans are non-indifferent to the environment. That is, they are part of the process by means of which humans adapt to and adjust the environment. One aspect of this process is the incorporation of technologies. However, another important aspect by means of which human beings exercise normativity is in technologically adjusting the environment. It is at this point that Canguilhem's account of health and the postphenomenological approach to technologies intersect. In *Technology and the Lifeworld*, Ihde notes that "it might be possible for humans to live non-technologically as a kind of abstract possibility—but only on the condition that the environment be that of a garden, isolated, protected, and stable" (Ihde, 1990, p.13). However, and this is what Canguilhem's analysis aptly shows, the environment in which we live does not resemble a stable garden. Rather, the environment is something inducing problematisation, and technological adjustment is a particular way of problematising the demands the environment puts on us.

Recall that Canguilhem defines the experience of health as the margin of tolerance for the inconstancies of the environment. The examples of everyday cyborg technologies point to the fact that it similarly consists of a margin of tolerance for the technologies that are being incorporated, and which, in turn constitute an environment in which new inconstancies emerge. Hence, as a result of the dynamic relationship between organism and environment, the milieus in which human beings live are constantly changing. Moreover, the idea of adaptation is crucial for Canguilhem's understanding of health, which presupposes that organisms never merge with an environment; they would either cease to exist when doing so, or make them unable to tolerate the aggressions of a multiplicity of environments that the organism will inevitably face.

However, as the discussion of technological incorporation in this chapter indicates, there seem to be many instances in which the boundaries between human organisms and the environment are unclear. In many cases, it becomes increasingly unclear where the organism "ends" and the environment "begins". And this lack of clarity is further complicated by the fact that the environment is one that is the result of the organism's activity. Following Canguilhem, it is fruitful to understand this lack of clarity experientially in that it fuels the human organism's norm-setting activity, such that the experience of being able to problematise is part of the experience of being healthy.

In the next chapter, I focus on a particular way in which health is problematised, namely through the discourse around personalised medicine, which I will treat as a specific case of turning medicine from a curative into a preventive endeavour. Technologies are thought to be key in realising the key aim of personalised medicine: they are thought to contribute to developing forms of self-governance that enable people to take better care of their own health. In what sense does personalised medicine indeed help the realisation of self-governance in the sense that it enables problematisation? And in what sense does it demand the coincidence with a particular kind of environment and/or with a particular set of (social) norms?

Notes

1 The notion of "disabled" carries some problematic assumptions with regard to the existence of some universal standard of "ability". While being aware of these assumptions and that the term "disabled" is sometimes contested, I have chosen to use the term in the context of this chapter as it is used by many researchers arguing for the acknowledgement of the everyday cyborg.

2 See also section 1.2.1

3 Canguilhem was one of Foucault's most important mentors. However, whereas Foucault has for long been a common point of reference in the English-speaking

world, it is only in the past two decades that the importance of Canguilhem's work in the philosophy of medicine and the philosophy of biology has been recognised outside of France.

References

Besmer, K. (2012). Embodying a translation technology: The cochlear implant and cyborg intentionality. *Techné: Research in Philosophy and Technology*, *16*(3), 296–316. https://doi.org/10.5840/techne201216319

Besmer, K. (2015). What robotic re-embodiment reveals about virtual re-embodiment. In R. Rosenberger & P.P-. Verbeek (Eds.), *Postphenomenoloigcal investigations: Essays on human-technology relations* (pp. 55–69). Lexington Books.

de Boer, B., Kudina, O., & Hoek, J. (2018). Can the technological mediation approach improve technology assessment? A critical view from 'within'. *Journal of Responsible Innovation*, *5*(3), 299–315. https://doi.org/10.1080/23299460.2018.1495029

de Boer, B., Te Molder, H., & Verbeek, P.P-. (2020). Constituting 'visual attention': On the mediating role of brain stimulation and brain imaging technologies in neuroscientific practice. *Science as Culture*, *29*(4), 503–523. https://doi.org/10.1080/09505431.2019.1710739

Canguilhem, G. (1991). *The normal and the pathological* (C.R. Fawcett, trans.). ZONE Books.

Canguilhem, G. (2012). *Writings on medicine* (S. Geroulanos & T. Meyers, trans.). Fordham University Press.

Clynes, M.E., & Kline, N.S. (1960). Cyborgs and space. *Astronautics*, *5*(9), 26–27, 24–76.

Coeckelbergh, M. (2017). *New romantic cyborgs: Romanticism, information technology, and the end of the machine*. The MIT Press.

Cromby, J., & Standen, P. (1999). Cyborgs and stigma: Technology, disability, subjectivity. In A. Gordo-Lopez & I. Parker (Eds.), *Cyberpsychology* (pp. 95–112). Routledge.

Forss, A. (2012). Cells and the (imaginary) patient: The multistable practitioner-technology-cell interface in the cytology laboratory. *Medicine, Health Care and Philosophy*, *15*, 295–308. https://doi.org/10.1007/s11019-011-9325-0

Goldstein, K. (1995). *The organism: A holistic approach to biology derived from pathological data in man*. Zone Books.

Haraway, D. (2016). *Manifestly Haraway*. The University of Minnesota Press.

Hayles, K. (1999). *How we became posthuman: Virtual bodies in cybernetics, literature and informatics*. University of Chicago Press.

Ihde, D. (1979). *Technics and praxis*. D. Reidel Publishing.

Ihde, D. (1990). *Technology and the lifeworld: From garden to earth*. Indiana University Press.

Ihde, D. (2002). *Bodies in technology*. The University of Minnesota Press.

Ihde, D. (2010). *Embodied technics*. Automatic Press.

Ihde, D. (2012). Postphenomenological re-embodiment. *Foundations of Science*, *17*, 373–377. https://doi.org/10.1007/s10699-011-9244-9

Kline, R. (2009). Where are the cyborgs in cybernetics? *Social Studies of Science*, *39*(3), 331–362. https://doi.org/10.1177/0306312708101046

Leder, D. (1990). *The absent body*. The University of Chicago Press.

Merleau-Ponty, M. (2012). *Phenomenology of perception* (D.A. Landes, trans.). Routledge.
Oudshoorn, N. (2020). *Resilient cyborgs: Living and dying with pacemakers and defibrillators*. Palgrave Macmillan.
Reeve, D. (2012). Cyborgs, cripples and iCrip: Reflections on the contribution of Haraway to disability studies. In D. Goodley, B. Hughes, & L.J. Davis (Eds.), *Disability and social theory: New developments and directions* (pp. 91–111). Palgrave Macmillan.
Rosenberger, R. (2012). Embodied technology and the dangers of using the phone while driving. *Phenomenology & the Cognitive Sciences*, *11*, 79–94. https://doi.org/10.1007/s11097-011-9230-2
Shew, A. (2020). From a figment of your imagination: Disabled marginal cases and underthought experiments. *Human Affairs*, *30*, 608–616. https://doi.org/10.1515/humaff-2020-0054
Sholl, J. (2016). Contextualizing medical norms: Georges Canguilhem's surnaturalism. In É. Giroux (Ed.), Naturalism in the philosophy of health (pp. 81-100). Springer.
Trnka, P. (2003). Subjectivity and values in medicine: The case of Canguilhem. *Journal of Medicine and Philosophy*, *28*(4), 427-446. https://doi.org/10.1076/jmep.28.4.427.15966
Van Den Eede, Y. (2011). In between us: On the transparency and opacity of technological mediation. *Foundations of Science*, *16*, 139–159. https://doi.org/10.1007/s10699-010-9190-y
Verbeek, P.P-. (2005). *What things do: Philosophical reflections on technology, agency, and design* (R.P. Crease, trans.). The State University of Pennsylvania Press.
Verbeek, P.P-. (2008). Cyborg intentionality: Rethinking the phenomenology of human-technology relations. *Phenomenology & the Cognitive Sciences*, *7*, 387–395. https://doi.org/10.1007/s11097-008-9099-x
Wellner, G. (2020). Postphenomenology of augmented reality. In H. Wiltse (Ed.), *Relating to things: Design, technology and the artificial* (pp. 173–187). Bloomsbury.

5 Personalised Medicine and Healthy Embodiment

Introduction

In many countries—especially Western countries—we have witnessed a specific problematisation of medicine in the last couple of decades. This problematisation involves two complementary imaginaries: (1) that medicine should become personalised medicine,[1] and (2) that this transformation enables to turn medicine from a curative into a preventive endeavour. The realisation of those imaginaries is thought to positively contribute to the health of individuals. Personalisation, on the one hand, is thought to enable the provision of better-tailored diagnostics and treatment. On the other hand, it allegedly also increases the ability of individuals to take control and responsibility for their own health by acting upon tailor-made lifestyle suggestions. This latter point reveals the close connection between personalised and preventive medicine: lifestyle changes are thought to be necessary to mitigate the occurrence of future diseases, thereby improving the health of individuals.

In this chapter, I propose to understand personalised medicine as a *sociotechnical imaginary* (Jasanoff, 2015). That is, even though it is far from evident that its ideals are practically realised or can be realised in the near future, it contains a vision of a desirable future grounded in the perceived potentialities of technoscience that people can collectively work towards. On a general level, the imaginaries of personalisation and prevention serve as potential solutions to the financial burden put on healthcare systems as a result of a growing elderly population; disease prevention through personalisation here is a means to ensure that people continue to have access to care in the (near) future. The success of these imaginaries is often framed in terms of how personalisation can help prevent future diseases by changing the lifestyle choices of individuals. Currently, this often depends on the active participation of people who collect health-related data about their own lives through practices of self-tracking. This marks a difference with earlier practices such as vaccination programmes (although this has become very topical again in recent years) or measures for ensuring clean

DOI: 10.4324/9781003602385-6

drinking water. These either involve environmental interventions or interventions that are not dependent on personalised and customised data. Another distinctive feature of the current imaginary of personalised medicine is that its success is dependent on the willingness of people to voluntarily change their behaviour and/or actively make lifestyle changes that are beneficial for their health; for example, abstaining from certain behaviours (e.g., overeating, alcohol use), or more frequently engaging in others (e.g., physical activity).

The implicit assumption underlying this understanding of personalised medicine seems to be that the behaviour and lifestyle of individuals are generally to be considered as risks that potentially undermine their health status. This idea of individuals always being-at-risk results in the production of a particular kind of subject that needs to be protected and/or needs to protect itself against influences that have a negative influence on their health. As we will see in this chapter, the imaginary of personalised medicine conceives of this being-at-risk in two different ways: on the one hand, it promotes an ideal of increasing precision that enables to outline the risks that individuals are subject to in molecular detail. On the other hand, it suggests that individuals need to change their behaviour or be empowered in order to better cope with the risks that they are subject to.

As we will see in this chapter, technological developments are thought to be key for the vision of personalised medicine. First of all, because they are thought to enable more detailed measurements of the physiological and molecular status of individuals that might result in diagnoses and treatments that are better tailored to the needs of individuals. And second, because technologies can be developed that enable to visualise data of relevant parameters, which allegedly enables users to get a better grip on how their behaviour or general lifestyle affects their health status. In tandem, then, these technological developments are taken to empower people to take better care of their health such that they are better able to face the risks that they are inevitably subjected to.

The goal of this chapter is to analyse how the imaginary of personalised medicine shapes the experience of healthy embodiment by applying the conceptual vocabulary developed in the previous chapter. The chapter is structured as follows: first, I introduce the key aspects of the ideal of personalised medicine and critically scrutinise to what extent it should be understood as a hype (Abettan, 2016). Second, I propose to understand personalised medicine as a sociotechnical imaginary, implying that regardless of whether it has been realised in practice, it has normative import because it provides a blueprint of which behaviours are desirable in light of the possible realisation of the imagined future, as well as in that there is a certain institutional pressure on people to help realising this future. Third, I analyse to what extent one of the central promises of personalised medicine, that of empowerment, indeed enables people to take better care of their own health. Finally, I discuss how the norms introduced by the sociotechnical imaginary of personalised medicine shape the experience of healthy embodiment in terms of how it enables new forms of problematisation.

§5.1 Personalised Medicine: What's in a Name?

A good starting point for understanding the aims and goals of personalised medicine are policy documents formulating its ideal. For instance, the Genomics and Personalised Medicine Act introduced by Barack Obama in 2007, when he was a senator from Illinois, provides the following definition: "Personalised medicine is the application of genomic and molecular data to better target the delivery of health care, facilitate the discovery and clinical testing of new products, and help determine a patient's predisposition to a particular disease or condition" (2007). In 2015, Obama shifted terminology and launched the Precision Medicine Initiative, where precision medicine is taken to be "an innovative approach that takes into account individual differences in people's genes, environments and lifestyles". This approach will eventually, so the initiative suggests, "enable healthcare provides to tailor treatment and prevention strategies to people's unique characteristics, including their genome sequence, microbiome composition, health history, lifestyle, and diet" (Precision Medicine Initiative, 2015). The European Council offers a slightly different perspective. While noting that there is no commonly accepted definition, they maintain that personalised medicine is widely understood as

> "a medical model using characterisation of individuals' phenotypes and genotypes (e.g., molecular profiling, medical imaging, lifestyle data) for tailoring the right therapeutic strategy for the right person at the right time, and/or to determine the predisposition to disease and/or to deliver timely and targeted prevention. Personalized medicine is related to the broader concept of patient-centred care."
>
> (European Council, 2015, p. 1)

From these varying definitions, we can derive that personalised medicine is far from a stable signifier and that there are no well-established boundaries between personalised medicine, precision medicine, patient-centred care and other terms such as participatory medicine or stratified medicine. Second, that there is a close relationship between personalised medicine and the prevention of disease, resulting in a situation in which public health and clinical medicine increasingly start fusing. Third, personalised medicine does not only focus on the inner functioning of the body but also intends to understand health and disease in terms of environmental and lifestyle factors. Lastly, medicine is understood as an increasingly data-intensive enterprise and made reliant on the availability of technologies that enable to monitor environmental and lifestyle factors, as well as on the ability and willingness of people to participate in such self-tracking practices. The overarching suggestion is that personalised medicine will cause a disruption in existing healthcare practice, and that turning medicine from a curative into a preventive practice, and more effective and individualised treatment and prevention, are much-needed responses to a population growing increasingly order and which puts financial pressure on existing healthcare systems and practices.

§5.1.1 The Disruption of Personalised Medicine: A Hype?

A very common response to proponents of personalised medicine that enthusiastically emphasise its disruptive potential, is: has it not been the goal of medicine from its inception to be personalised? Although the language might have been slightly different, also Ayurvedic practices around 4000 BC and Hippocrates' writings seem to suggest that medicine is about the treatment of individual patients whose health and illness cannot be understood in general terms (Cesario et al., 2021). Or, another indication can be found in Aristotle's *Metaphysics*, where he writes: "the physician does not cure a man, except in an incidental way, but Callias or Socrates or some other called by some such individual name, who happens to be a man" (Metaphysics, 981a, 19–20). The ideal of medicine as targeting specific individuals that cannot be reduced to general characteristics is thus far from new.

However, that medicine has had an ideal of personalisation throughout its long history does of course not necessarily imply that it was close to realising this ideal. It is in this regard that proponents of personalised medicine typically position themselves in relation to earlier forms of medical practice. While acknowledging continuity throughout history in terms of the ideal of medicine, these proponents typically posit that there was an epistemological and technological deficit when it comes to the possibility of coming close to realising this ideal. It is thought that only after the development of the -omics sciences from the mid-20th century onwards and the possibility to systematically collect and organise relevant health-related data that the notion of personalised medicine can be meaningfully operationalised.[2]

If one intends to evaluate the promise of personalised medicine, the question is if the -omics sciences and the collection of health-related data do indeed contribute to personalisation, as well as how the notion of personalisation is generally understood. Gamma (2017, p. 397) distinguishes between two understandings of personalised medicine: a broader view that takes more or less any feature of an individual (be it environmental, biological, or psychological) as relevant for decision-making when it comes to treatment and prevention, and a more narrow view that essentially considers molecular biology and the individual's genetic make-up as the key to personalisation. According to Gamma, it is the latter view that corresponds to how personalised medicine is actually practised, such that it is this operationalisation of the ideal that should be scrutinised.

Gamma further argues that, insofar as personalised medicine is grounded in the idea that the gene should be the central unit of investigation, it most likely will not be of much clinical value, since "most illnesses are determined by a complex interplay of genetic and non-genetic factors" (Gamma, 2017, p. 400). Personalised medicine is trapped in a mistaken understanding of genes that can be dubbed the information metaphor, according to which genes carry information that should be understood as instructions controlling the development of individual organisms. This understanding of genes takes them to be the most relevant causal factors for health or disease. However, as Gamma points out, almost without exception, most studies on genes undermine the tenability of this metaphor, such that they should not be understood as "privileged origins of disease nor [as] privileged intervention points" (Gamma, 2017, p. 402). Or, put differently, a form of reductionism that takes genes to be offering the ultimate explanation of health and illness is bound to miss the mark. Even if the most up-to-date science would be able to give a complete picture of the genetic make-up of each individual patient, this would not be sufficient to provide an adequate marker for health and illness as it neglects relevant environmental, psychological and social factors. This makes that Gamma comes to a rather bleak evaluation of personalised medicine: insofar as it is driven by the information metaphor, it should be considered a hype with little relevance for how medicine is and/or should be practised.

The irreducibility of health and illness to one's genetic make-up is well-recognised by medical professionals and biomedical researchers. For instance, Pokorska-Bocci and colleagues argue that personalised medicine must not be understood as a

> technocratic replacement for clinical judgment mostly based on advances in genomic medicine, but as a complex endeavor with a holistic lifetime approach in which both healthcare providers and individual healthcare users, in active partnership, take full advantage of the portfolio of modern tools and information available.
>
> (Pokorska-Bocci et al., 2014, p. 207)

An earlier anonymous critical evaluation of personalised medicine argued that "patients—and ultimately all individuals—will need to be educated about the benefits of a healthy lifestyle and wellness and disease prevention. Government plans [...] will help, but new technologies should be made available that help patients monitor their health, share their medical data and seek attention when needed" (Anonymous, 2012, p. 1). Such interventions assume that the (bio-)medical sciences can offer all kinds of relevant information when it comes to healthy lifestyles and diets, as well as one's predisposition to develop specific diseases, but that patients and healthcare providers should cooperate in finding out how this information can be made relevant for individuals and be acted upon. On such a view, personalised medicine itself is not necessarily a hype or empty fantasy, but needs to develop in a different direction in order to live up to its initial expectations.

Such a conception is in line with Gamma's broader understanding of personalised medicine in which more or less any feature of an individual becomes relevant for treatment or intervention. If indeed almost all aspects of an individual—including the structure of their everyday lives—should become part of the project of personalised medicine, it is crucial that people are able and willing to voluntarily collect and share massive amounts of data (e.g., about their nutrition, lifestyle, physical activities), that it is possible to link this data to relevant markers of health and illness (i.e., that the technologies to do so are available), and that this data can be made actionable. Vogt and colleagues describe this development in terms of a holistic medicalisation that has moved beyond a hope of controlling "disease by manipulating of a few factors to hoping to control [disease] through management of the whole, dynamic life process" (2016, p. 321), resulting in a medicalisation of life itself. Bearing in mind the lessons of Chapters 2 and 3, the next section asks to what extent such a fear of "total medicalisation" is justified by focusing on how the data-intensive practice of personalised medicine constitute a particular kind of subjectivity. This will be done by introducing the notion of *sociotechnical imaginary*, which will prove useful in theorising how personalised medicine can be understood as constituting subjectivity, despite it being to a large extent a hype that is far from realised.

§5.2 Personalised Medicine as a Sociotechnical Imaginary

Personalised medicine confronts us with a puzzling situation. On the one hand, many researchers—both in the medical sciences and those having a critical approach to medicine—recognise that personalised medicine fails to live up to its initial hype, such that it is almost meaningless to speak of it as relevantly informing clinical practice. On the other hand, it seems that although the results of personalised medicine have not had much of a bearing on clinical practice, people in general are certainly willing to engage in data-collecting practices that they deem to be relevant for their health. The latter issue results in a fear of the medicalisation of life proper and an according questioning of the practice of tracking data for health-related purposes.

The notion of *sociotechnical imaginary* as developed by Jasanoff and Kim helps explain this situation. Jasanoff defines sociotechnical imaginaries as "collectively held, institutionally stabilised, and publicly performed visions of desirable futures, animated by shared understandings of forms of social life and social order attainable through, and supportive of, advances in science and technology" (Jasanoff, 2015, p. 4).[3] While crucially interrelated with technoscientific developments, such imaginaries not only contain visions of "what is attainable through science and technology but also of how life ought, or ought not, to be lived; in this respect they express a society's shared understandings of good and evil" (Jasanoff, 2015, p. 4). Sociotechnical imaginaries are thus inspired by the perceived potentialities of technoscience that are thought to imagine a desirable future that people can collectively work towards when behaving in a certain manner. This vision of an imagined future, then, has normative import in that it provides a blueprint of which behaviours are desirable in light of the possible realisation of the imagined future, as well as in that there is a certain institutional pressure on people to help realising this future.

It is worthwhile to emphasise that "imaginary" is not used a pejorative concept and implies a dismissive value judgement, referring something utterly unrealistic or a free-floating fantasy. Of course, imaginaries might be partly unrealistic or rich in fantasy. However, what ultimately characterises imaginaries is that they provide a vision of what reality should look like or of what kind of order should emerge, which materialises even if it does contain certain aspects of this vision do, strictly speaking, not become tangible. Hence, even if personalised medicine cannot live up to its initial promise or hype, it does remain circumscribing what kinds of lives or behaviours are taken to be desirable.

Jasanoff explicitly positions herself in relation to Foucault: "[A]s Foucault pre-eminently observed, when bodies are well disciplined to live inside those orders, what looks natural from on high may not be so different from what looks natural from below. The same collective imaginary may condition and constrain the sense of justice that binds a community" (Jasanoff, 2015, p. 14). Sociotechnical imaginaries, in line with Foucault's thought, function to discipline bodies in a certain manner and induce specific practices of care that are shaped by the imagined future within a certain collective. It is in this sense, that sociotechnical imaginaries embody a specific logic of power in that they constitute a particular form of subjectivity that needs to be sustained for the desirable future to remain attainable.

Tutton takes the "imaginary of personalised medicine to refer to the speculative, propositional fabric of scientific thought concerned with the application of genomic knowledge and technologies to the biomedical enterprise" (Tutton, 2014, p. 10). As we saw in the previous section, initiatives like the Precision Medicine Initiative or the efforts by the European Commission flesh out in what sense this application provides a desirable future: personalised medicine is described as a future in which more targeted care is realised and in which the number of hospital visits decreases through targeted prevention. This is taken to be both an answer to increasing financial pressures on many (Western) healthcare systems and a way to maintain an ideal of a healthy population that is potentially under threat by "lifestyle-related diseases".

Let me now explain in more detail in what sense personalised medicine specifically can be considered as a sociotechnical imaginary. To do so, it is helpful to break up Jasanoff's (2015) definition into its individual components. This enables us to illustrate the extent that personalised medicine is a vision that is (1) attainable through and supportive of advances in science and technology, (2) institutionally stabilised, (3) publicly performed, (4) collectively held and (5) animates shared understanding of social life and social order.

Developments in the -omics sciences, as well as in the accuracy and availability of sensor and tracking technologies, are thought to be key reservoirs for the realisation of personalised medicine. As we saw, on the one hand, an increase in knowledge of people's genetic make-up and molecular processes are thought to be the key to personalisation. On the other hand, the ideal of personalisation is further fuelled by the ubiquitous availability of technologies that enable the tracking of increasingly many aspects of the daily lives of people. And even if technoscience does not enable to fulfil the aims of personalisation yet, it is thought of as holding the promise of realising those aims in the future. This is why there remains an ongoing interest in funding technoscientific initiatives claiming to work towards personalisation, even if they have thus far not proven to be relevant to clinical practice.

The institutional stabilisation of personalised medicine can be exemplified by the presence of specific funding structures as well as the establishment of political initiatives. Funding structures, especially those oriented to creating research consortia in which large groups of researchers are brought together, provide an opportunity to collaborate on topics related to personalised medicine for longer periods of time. In this way, the continuity of researchers publishing on relevant topics and the organisation of conferences around those is maintained. These can be considered to be activities that have an important function in terms of agenda-setting, such that the topic of personalised medicine remains visible to politicians and its promise(s) remain being communicated. Moreover, developments such as the passing of the Genomics and Personalised Medicine Act in the USA in 2007, as well as initiatives on the European continent, such as the 2018 Dutch national health prevention act, ensure continuity by formulating a vision for politicians and/or ministries of health that they can be held accountable for.

The vision of personalised medicine is further stabilised by the support of public figures. For instance, visible public figures such as Barack Obama or Bill Gates actively support, provide funding, or even establish research institutes related to the development of medicine into a preventive and personalised endeavour. Moreover, medical professionals regularly appear in newspapers, online, or on television to highlight the potential benefits of personalised medicine and stress the need for using technologies enabling to work towards leading a "healthy lifestyle" (e.g., Lewis, 2008; Petersen, 2019). Besides, the massive presence and interest in commercial self-tracking devices (e.g., smartwatches, diet trackers, mobile self-tracking applications) is also indicative of the public performance of the vision of imaginary medicine. For instance, the availability of commercials and billboards by means of which tech companies (e.g., Apple, Samsung) advertise products relevant to health-tracking, as well as the general increasing visibility of these products when people use them.

Explaining if and how personalised medicine is grounded in collectively held assumptions about health and medicine and might animate a shared understanding of social life and social order requires a more sophisticated analysis that will be carried out in the next subsection. The widespread use of health-tracking technologies and the ongoing funding towards biomedical research related to personalisation suggest that both political institutions and individuals generally collectively hold the assumption that personalised medicine constitutes a desirable future. However, the presence of these phenomena is in itself not sufficient to show that there is indeed something shared across the different people engaging in activities related to personalisation. This requires establishing a link between sociotechnical imaginaries and subjectification.

§5.2.1 *Life as Sickness unto Death: Everyone Patient?*

> The physician knows that just as there is merely imaginary sickness, there is also merely imaginary health, and in the latter case he first takes measures to disclose the sickness.
>
> (Kierkegaard, 1980 [1849], p. 23).

This quote by Kierkegaard, although pulled a bit out of context, nicely illustrates the rationale behind personalised medicine. Its main idea is that the majority of the population acts as if they are healthy and even experience themselves as healthy, whereas they actually carry all kinds of diseases or are at risk of getting (severely) ill in the near future. Or, framed in terms of the title of Kierkegaard's book: life is a sickness unto death. And even though this title had, for Kierkegaard, no direct bearing on the medical sciences proper, the idea that underlying our smooth everyday experience there is something slumbering that can awaken every moment seems very much in line with how personalised medicine is promoted and legitimated.

In fact, since personalised medicine is highly data-driven, "[w]ithout patients contributing data, time, effort and self-care, current visions of personalized medicine cannot be realized" (Prainsack, 2017, p. 11). It is therefore critical that (prospective) patients and people more generally maintain that it is worthwhile to contribute to practices of data-gathering, either because they believe that this data is relevant for treating their illness, or because they think that this data is indeed indicative of the slumbering sickness that is explicitly or tacitly present in their lives, such that preventive measures are needed.

Related to the above, the vision of personalised medicine "is not only a matter of change in institutional and professional practice but also a profound change in the sick role" (Strand, 2022, p. 313). Whereas the sick role, a term taken from Parsons (1951), previously related to the responsibilities of individuals to actively seek treatment and follow medical procedures needed for them to be recognised as sick, the vision of personalised medicine introduces novel expectations: it requires people experiencing illness that they actively contribute to medical decision-making by collecting data on aspects of their body and everyday life that doctors deem relevant and by sharing this data with medical professionals. But, on top of this, the focus on targeted prevention also asks people that were initially classified as healthy or who experience themselves as healthy to adopt a similar sick role, in that they also need to be willing to collect data about everyday activities and display a willingness to change aspects of their everyday lives for future health gains.

This aspect enables to emphasise another feature of sociotechnical imaginaries, namely that it produces a particular kind of subject that is supposed to engage in a particular kind of conduct. In Jasanoff's words, "elements of human subjectivity and agency get bound up with technoscientific advances through adjustments in identities, institutions, and discourses that accompany new representations of things" (2015, p.14). By introducing a new range of phenomena as being representative of health and illness and explicitly transforming these concepts from referring to the present as ones referring to future states of affairs, subjectivity is shaped in that humans are invited to ongoingly take care of themselves and their bodies to decrease the risk of being unhealthy.

Many researchers in science and technology studies (STS) have pointed to how personalised medicine shapes how humans understand themselves. Some analyses echo Illich's criticism of medicine developed in *Medical Nemesis* in that they similarly argue that personalised medicine prevents human beings from coming to grips with their own finitude (e.g.,

Blasimme, 2017; Strand, 2022). This, so such authors maintain, prevents people from developing a vision on the good life, which is why personalised medicine can be considered to be ethically harmful. However, as we saw in chapter 2, while worthwhile, such criticisms too easily discard the productive capacity of subjects, and implicitly presuppose power to be unidirectionally flowing from medical institutions to citizens. However, if sociotechnical imaginaries are productive of subjectivity, such a unidirectional understanding misses the mark, in that subjectivity always implies that people remain capable of positioning themselves in relation to power structures.

Other analyses are more in line with the account of power inspired by Foucault that guides the analysis of this book. For instance, Abettan and Weile recognise that "personalization of medicine is not considered the result of tailoring health care to the uniqueness of a pre-existing person. Rather, the process of personalization itself (by which the person is becoming who he/she is) occurs—at least in part—on the basis of all the data disclosed by personalized medicine" (Abettan & Weile, 2020, p. 2). On such a view, personalisation does not extract data from a pre-existing human being that subsequently attains a better understanding of who it has always been but instead produces a novel human during the process of tailoring.

Chiapperino and Testa (2016) even go so far as to say that a new epigenomic self is created through the shift towards personalised medicine. This self emerges as a result of two interrelated developments: the rise of molecular epigenomics and the discourse of empowerment accompanying healthcare changes instantiated by personalisation. On the one hand, the sociotechnical imaginary of personalised medicine is grounded in the promise of an increase in knowledge of the body's functioning and genetic make-up made possible by technoscientific developments. On the other hand, so Chiapperino and Testa maintain, the promissory discourse simultaneously catalyses demands and expectations on citizens (2016, p. 204). That is, through the availability of knowledge, people are expected to take care of themselves in terms of the promises of personalised medicine by regularly participating in activities such as preventive screening, acting upon the knowledge acquainted by means of such activities, and shape their everyday lives in terms of it. The discourse of empowerment, then, asks citizens to engage in a specific form of self-governance resulting in a particular kind of "healthy" conduct.

It is because of this demand to put oneself under a certain governmental regime that critical scholars argue that personalised medicine—just as other technoscientific developments—is constitutive of subjectivity. And since this produced subject is supposed to spend increasingly more time on health-related activities that help preventing future illnesses from occurring, individuals who were previously considered to be healthy—living in the silence of the organs, as Canguilhem would have it—are constituted as patients who have to explicitly position themselves in relation to their slumbering illnesses and are expected to care for those.

The way this subjectivity is constituted cannot, as will be elaborated in the next section, be cut loose from the process by means of which medical knowledge is gathered. As we will see, the expectations and demands catalysed by personalised medicine are contingent on how people are made part of a particular population; a process shaping what are considered to be desirable forms of self-governance.

§5.3 The Population of Personalised Medicine and the Ideal of Empowerment

In what sense does personalised medicine understand bodies to be part of a population? Doesn't the very notion of personalisation presuppose a vision in which medicine will be grounded in the unique characteristics of (prospective) patients? In describing the history of medicine's recent efforts at precision and personalisation, Philips shows that "the ability to predict how a 'given treatment will affect a given individual' consequently relies—somewhat ironically—upon a history of *aggregating* patient data alongside measurements of therapeutic outcomes" (Philips, 2020, p. 4). And Tutton (2014, p. 167) suggests that personalised medicine has always revolved around two related but distinct narratives, namely the customisation of knowledge to individuals (e.g., targeted pharmaceuticals) and the empowerment of individuals to manage their own health risks. Both of those narratives are related in that they both present personalised medicine as a way to manage the slumbering illnesses present in human bodies and to enable individuals to calculate future health risks. Doing so necessarily presupposes the idea of a population that introduces a standard of normality from which deviations can be interpreted in terms of risks.

Élodie Giroux (2020, 2021) tries to reconcile the universalising and personalising tendencies of contemporary medicine through a critical appreciation of Canguilhem's work and argues that the notion of population, or population health, is indispensable for understanding individual health. This suggests that personalised medicine can shape the qualitative experience of health central in Canguilhem's account. Recall that for Canguilhem, health is a concept only applying to the individual and that applying the term to populations or societies should be considered purely metaphorical. Health, for Canguilhem, is the qualitative expression of biological normativity on the level of the individual. And since a population can only exist in terms of quantitative statistical variations, it cannot offer an indication of the health of individuals. At the same time, as we saw, Canguilhem recognises that societal norms around health shape how we understand ourselves and our health status. As he puts it, being healthy implies not only to live life "in the silence of the organs—it is also life lived in the discretion of social relations. If I say [...] that I am unwell, people want to know how and why; they wonder or ask me whether I am registered with social security" (Canguilhem, 2012, pp. 49–50).

Whereas Canguilhem dismisses that institutional aspects of medicine such as social security should have a bearing on individual health and hence on clinical medicine, Giroux argues that this dismissal is a relic of the past in that it is grounded in a distinction between clinical medicine and public health that is no longer tenable. As a result of this distinction, she maintains, "we perceive individual health and population health as two independent realities. But [...] the two are tightly interdependent such that clinical medicine and public health must work together. The trajectory of population health interacts with that of each individual" (Giroux, 2020, p. 73).

And insofar public health aims to contribute to empowerment, it becomes immediately clear how interventions on a population level have a bearing on the individual experience of health and vice versa. The World Health Organisation defines empowerment as "a process through which people gain greater control over decisions and actions affecting their health" (2021, p. 14). Hence, empowerment allegedly helps people to gain control over many factors in their lives that are relevant to their health, but which currently are not or cannot be (immediately) utilised, and health promotion is thought to contribute to the realisation of this ideal (Cyril, Smith & Renzaho, 2016).

§5.3.1 *The Uneasy Relationship between Personalised Medicine and Empowerment*

To start understanding what the notion of empowerment entails, it is helpful to distinguish it from what can be called the behaviour change approach in the context of personalised medicine.[4] The behaviour change approach in health promotion searches to influence people to change specific health-related behaviours (e.g., stop smoking, exercise more, use bike helmets) that allegedly have a negative effect on health (Laverack, 2017; Tengland, 2012, 2016). In this approach, it is pre-defined what constitutes "healthy behavior", and the main task is to make the behaviour of individuals align with this ideal. Hence, the specific interventions developed within this approach and the theories and models that they build upon are *instrumental* means to reach a specific goal. Individuals engaging in a particular kind of unhealthy behaviour, then, are conceptualised as having certain psychological characteristics (e.g., beliefs, desires, attitudes, self-efficacy) that are taken to be in need of correction through specific interventions (Tengland, 2012, p. 142). For example, making someone refrain from smoking cigarettes can be done through educating individuals about the harms of smoking, minimising one's desire to smoke, promoting a specific negative attitude towards smoking and smokers, or increasing one's self-control in order to be able to suppress one's urge for a cigarette.

However, the behaviour change approach problematically assumes that (1) health professionals know (better than the individuals they target) what *should* be the goals and interests one should pursue, and (2) that health interventions should focus on the behaviour and psychology of individuals, instead of considering health to be a collective problem (e.g., Goldberg, 2012). The former assumption is deemed to be problematic because it contradicts the common intuition that being healthy also crucially involves being able to set one's own goals and trying to achieve them. A top-down approach that imposes certain goals onto individuals as being the ultimately desirable ones might thus go at the expense of what individuals find important themselves. This results in a kind of health that is endorsed by others (doctors, health professionals, care providers, governments) but not necessarily experienced by the individual in question as healthy for them. If this common intuition is correct, then this top-down approach is problematic because it goes against one of the core components of being healthy, namely the development and pursuit of goals that one has set for oneself and that reflect some degree of self-determination.

The second assumption is problematic because it turns being healthy into a problem at the level of the targeted individual. As has been argued in several studies, an important adverse effect of this focus is that it leads to stigmatisation and victim-blaming (e.g., Brewis & Wutich, 2019; Puhl & Heuer, 2009). Since targeting the individual assumes that someone is and should be well informed about the health risks of certain behaviours, the burden of not adopting recommended behaviours is put on the individual. For example, the blame for the effects of overeating is put on the individual who is allegedly too weak-willed (or otherwise being irresponsible), such that it is treated as an individual failure. However, overeating might be (and often is) influenced by factors that individuals have little control over, such as the presence of certain cultural food norms, the smart and effective advertisement of fast food, and the easy access to inexpensive fast food, making eating more expensive healthy food a less attractive or even unattainable option.

In conjunction, these two problems point to a form of normativity that remains unaddressed in the behaviour change approach: (1) health professionals themselves act as a source of normativity by rendering certain goals and interests as (un)desirable and (un)healthy, which do not have to correspond with what particular individuals consider to be desirable and (un)healthy; (2) the interests and goals of individuals are to a large extent influenced and possibly obstructed or violated by socio-economic forces and norms; these (unconsciously) structure and influence their behaviour.

The empowerment approach can be seen as an attempt to correct and/or supplement the behaviour change approach. Empowerment can be loosely defined as a state in which individuals or groups can exercise a large degree of control on relevant determinants of their quality of life (e.g., Tengland, 2016, p. 34). As a result, the empowerment approach to health promotion is specifically concerned with how individuals can start to set their own goals and follow their own norms. "Empowering", then, is the process through which this control can be obtained and exercised. The emphasis on having control contrasts with the behaviour change approach because being "empowered" presupposes the ability to set and pursue one's own goals, rather than goals predetermined by someone else, such as the government, society or health professionals.

As a goal of personalised medicine, "empowerment" thus refers to the implementation of those measures that help people increase their capacity to control relevant health determinants. Instead of intending to change a particular behavior, interventions that aim for empowerment have increased control itself as a primary goal and are primarily concerned with the promotion of a particular ability. What, then, is this particular ability in the context of one's health, and with regard to which determinants should one exercise control?

On Tengland's account, the crucial ability needed to attain control over the determinants for one's quality of life is *self-governance*: the ability of an individual to make decisions over her own life and act upon those (2016, p. 37). Instead of being concerned with changing the behaviour of individuals in order to be able to better fulfil predetermined goals, the empowerment approach is concerned with changing both the socio-economic circumstances in which individuals live and the development of skills that increase their ability of self-governance. Hence, empowerment also requires sufficient knowledge about what one's decisions entail, the societal and political context in which those decisions are executed, and the motivation to embark on them. Examples of these are access to basic healthcare, increasing literacy or promoting the ability to engage in family planning. For example, if a person decides to become a parent and raise two children and at the same time pursue a career, they are empowered when having increased control over the determinants that contribute to realising this. This requires, for example (financial) access to (day) care facilities for her children, awareness that such care facilities exist, adequate housing to raise children, or knowledge about which behaviours to avoid when being pregnant and the ability to act upon this.

However, since humans are always situated in an environment that imposes norms on them, they are never completely free in how to govern themselves, but also need to adapt to certain social and environmental norms. These norms are dependent on one's own bodily condition in relation to the environment (e.g., I cannot walk through a wall, or I will get ill or die when being exposed to extreme temperatures), are socially constituted (e.g., a good parent should behave in this way) or are a mixture of both (e.g., given your ability to take care of your material body, you should aim to reach a certain age). As the latter type of norms indicate, biomedicine and health promotion are normative and therefore play an important role in determining what is sick, normal and healthy (Hancock, 2018; Harvey, 2010). Complete coincidence with a particular (set of) norm(s) cannot be considered a form of empowerment, as this would imply that someone is governed by something external rather than engaging in *self-governance*. At the same time, one's ability to set one's own norms is always limited by things that are beyond one's control, as it is impossible to completely detach oneself from one's biological constitution or societal context. Accordingly, empowerment involves a tension between self-governance and adaptation, and hence reveals that insofar as empowerment is one of the goals of personalised medicine, it does not mean to comply with more stringent health norms and to participate in voluntary collecting and sharing data about health-related parameters. That is, whereas measures to empower people might originate in approaching individuals as part of a population, the concept of empowerment—which entails self-governance—at the same time shows that the individual experience of being empowered cannot be reduced to one being part of a particular population.

§5.4 Conclusion: Personalised Medicine, Problematisation and Health Empowerment

What we learn from the above analysis of empowerment is that the concept of empowerment crucially entails self-governance but, at the same time, we cannot cut this form of governance loose from the problematisation of health and medicine present in the sociotechnical imaginary of personalised medicine. This tension can be fruitfully framed in terms of Foucault's notions of counter-conduct and problematisation: em*power*ment implies to be able to position oneself in relation to the powers that one is subjected to and to problematise one's own conduct in terms of how one desires to be governed.[5]

The ideal of personalised medicine is, as we have seen, grounded in how medical professionals and policymakers problematise existing forms of medicine, as well as ways in which people take care of their own health. That is, it is a sociotechnical imaginary that intends to impose a particular conduct onto citizens, either by making them engage in certain activities (e.g., data-tracking, dieting) or by creating a disciplining infrastructure that invites certain conduct. On the one hand, empowerment can be understood in terms of conforming to this specific problematisation and becoming the disciplined—or docile—subject. On the other hand, as we saw, to be conducted implies problematising this exercise of power in terms of how one desires to be governed. In this context, problematisation can occur on two different levels: on the level of the physiologically and habitually constituted body that shapes the subject one is and which can become the target of problematisation, or on the level of one's body is part of a population that needs to be governed and which is institutionally constituted and which also can become a target of problematisation.

The first level of problematisation brings us back to some crucial aspects of Canguilhem's account of health discussed in the previous chapter. First, it is important to remain understanding empowerment as a form of problematisation as involving *bodily* experience. Taking a phenomenological starting point, the experience of being healthy involves that someone is not exclusively focusing on one's body, but instead is capable of using one's body to transcend into other projects (Carel, 2021). Experiencing one's body as hindrance to engage in projects in the environment, is a mark of being unable to tolerate and cope with the aggressions of the environment (Toro et al., 2020). This very experience constitutes a source for problematisation one's conduct. Second, Canguilhem helps reminding that the environment in which the organism lives is far from stable, both because the organism is inevitably in motion, constantly encountering new environments, and because any environment is partly constituted by the organism's own normative capacities. Hence, another way of problematisation consists in addressing one's the ability of not-coinciding with a particular environment amongst the *multiplicity* of environments that someone inevitably encounters.

Following Foucault, the next question is to what extent these to forms of problematisation must be interpreted in terms of governing one's own conduct. The problematisation of one's own bodily experience requires a governing of one's own conduct in relation to the projects one intends to carry out. Put differently, the environment is one that cannot be tolerated and coped with by the experiencing subject. For instance, when one experiences a mismatch between the projects that one desires to carry out and the capacity to actually pursue these projects, one can either govern oneself by formulating other projects and ideals or by targeting the limits of one's own body as in need of better governance. That is, one can problematise the experiential environment either in terms of how it is constituted by one's projects or in terms of how it is constituted by one's physiological and habitual constitution.

The problematisation of one's capacity to tolerate the aggression of a multiplicity of environments is more explicitly future-oriented. This form of problematisation is partly in line with the institutional goals of personalised medicine, as it is grounded in the idea that whereas one is currently able to unproblematically transcend into the world, this capacity might decline in the future. Therefore, what is problematised is the extent to which one's current conduct enables one to tolerate the aggressions of environments other than the one that an individual happens to be "in", and to find ways of governance that prevent that one is only able to be normative in one particular environment. For instance, one can problematise the existing habitual constitution of one's own body in light of the extent to which this constitution shapes the future possibility to exercise one's normativity.

A second level on which personalised medicine can give rise to problematisation is by challenging how the population of which one is a part is governed and problematised. That is, one might come up with alternative ways—that are not necessarily ingrained into the institutional ideal of personalised medicine—to use new medical developments for self-governance. Insofar as the sociotechnical imaginary can be considered to exercise power and to shape the conduct of individuals—and given the institutional environment and policy initiatives, it does not seem unreasonable to accept this, it gives, following Foucault, rise to counter-conduct that is grounded in the collective desire to be governed differently.

Also on this level, problematisations can have different targets. For instance, one can problematise the extent to which the ways of personalisation enabled by medical professionals have an actual bearing on one's life. Problematisation, here, targets the notion of population in that a discrepancy is experienced between what is personalised in terms of an aggregate within a specific group and in terms of one's own experience what is good for one's body. In this case, health-related data and the practice of personalisation are integrated into another governmental regime. Another way of problematising the population is not to question the extent of personalisation but rather that one belongs to a specific kind of population that is not sufficiently acknowledged in the current formulation of personalised medicine. This form of counter-conduct, then, orients to the constitution of a population that allegedly more adequately reflects on one's own bodily constitution.

The general aim of this chapter was to explore how personalised medicine can shape the embodied experience of health. In doing so, I have proposed to understand personalised medicine as a sociotechnical imaginary. When framing personalised medicine as a sociotechnical imaginary, it becomes clear that regardless of the extent to which it is practically realised, it does carry normative import by providing a blueprint of what healthy conduct should look like. This is because of it being primarily a professional and institutional initiative about how medical practice and health-related behaviour *should* be organised, thereby providing a direction into which societies should develop.

The extent to which this vision is realised or will be realised in the near future is questionable, and the shape that the vision will eventually take is unclear. In terms of Gamma's (2017) distinction, there is no clarity if personalised medicine in the end will have a more narrow biomedical understanding of personalisation focusing on expert interpretations of one's molecular biology and genetic make-up, or a broader view that takes more or less any feature of an individual (be it environmental, biological, or psychological) as relevant for decision-making when it comes to treatment and prevention, and which places more emphasis on the responsibility of individuals to develop specific lifestyles. The concrete development of personalised medicine is dependent on how health is problematised and turned into an object of government. The embodied experience of health is constituted relative to such problematisations, as are the practices of counter-conduct emerging from this experience.

Notes

1 There is no clear consensus on what exactly constitutes personalised medicine and how it can be distinguished from neighbouring concepts such as precision medicine, participatory medicine, or preventive medicine (see also section 5.3 of this chapter). To maintain conceptual continuity, I have decided to use—unless otherwise indicated—the notion of personalised medicine to refer to all efforts directed at preventing future diseases by making medicine better tailored to individuals.

2 The complex history of personalised medicine in the US and Great Britain is extensively discussed in Richard Tutton's *Genomics and the Reimagining of Personalized Medicine* (Tutton, 2014).

3 This 2015 definition slightly differs from the one initially proposed in 2009. Initially, sociotechnical imaginaries were defined as "collectively imagined form of social life and social order reflected in the design and fulfillment of nation-specific scientific and/or technological projects" (Jasanoff & Kim, 2009, p. 120). The most important novel elements for our purposes are that the new definition does not take sociotechnical imaginaries to be nation-specific and points to their relative degree of institutional stability. A detailed comparative discussion of these different definitions is beyond the scope of the present endeavour.

4 Although in practice, these two approaches are often not as clearly set apart, analytically distinguishing between them allows for revealing the different goals and strategies present in preventive medicine and health promotion.

5 I will refrain from describing the exact content of such problematisations as those will depend on the idiosyncrasies of the lives of specific individuals. Neither do I intend to provide an exhaustive list of possible problematisations. What I intend to point to is (a) that the power exercised by the sociotechnical imaginary of personalised medicine shapes the subjectivity of individuals in different ways, and (b) that these problematisations shape the experience of one's own body.

References

Abettan, C. (2016). Between hype and hope: What is really at stake with personalized medicine. *Medicine, Health Care and Philosophy*, *19*(3), 423–430. https://doi.org/10.1007/s11019-016-9697-2

Abettan, C., & Welie, J.V.M. (2020). The impact of twenty-first century personalized medicine versus twenty-first century medicine's impact on personalization. *Philosophy, Ethics, and Humanities in Medicine*, *15*, 11. https://doi.org/10.1186/s13010-020-00095-2

Anonymous. (2012). What happened to personalized medicine? *Nature Biotechnology*, *30*(1), 1. https://doi.org/10.1038/nbt.2096

Aristotle. (1985). Metaphysics. In J. Barnes (Ed.), *The complete works of Aristotle: Volume two* (pp. 1552–1728). Oxford University Press. (Original work published ca. 350 B.C.E.)

Blasimme, A. (2017). Health research meets big data: The science and politics of precision medicine. In A. Blanchard & R Strand (Eds.), *Cancer biomarkers: Ethics, economics and society* (pp. 95–109). Megacoleros Press.

Brewis, A., & Wutich, A. (2019). *Lazy, crazy and disgusting: Stigma and the undoing of global health*. John Hopkins University Press.

Canguilhem, G. (2012). *Writings on medicine* (S. Geroulanos & T. Meyers, trans.). Fordham University Press.

Carel, H. (2021). Pathology as a phenomenological tool. *Continental Philosophy Review*, *54*, 201–217. https://doi.org/10.1007/s11007-021-09538-9

Cesario, A., Lohmeyer, F.M., D'Oria, M., Manto, A., & Scambia, G. (2021). The personalized medicine discourse: Archeology and genealogy. *Medicine, Health Care and Philosophy*, *24*(2), 247–253. https://doi.org/s11019-020-09997-6

Chiapperino, L., & Testa, G. (2016). The epigenomic self in personalized medicine: Between responsibility and empowerment. *The Sociological Review*, *64*(1), 203–220. https://doi.org/10.1111/2059–7932.12021

Cyril, S., Smith, B.J., & Renzaho, A.M.N. (2016). Systematic review of empowerment measures in health promotion. *Health Promotion International*, *31*(4), 809–826. https://doi.org/10.1093/heapro/dav059

European Council. (2015). Council conclusions on personalised medicine for patients. *Official Journal of the European Union*, *431*, 1–4.

Gamma, A. (2017). Personalized and precision medicine. In M. Solomon, J.R. Simon, & H. Kincaid (Eds.), *The Routledge companion to philosophy of medicine* (pp. 397–407). Routledge.

Giroux, É. (2020). Is personalized medicine humanist? *Archives de Philosophie*, *83*(4), 59–82.

Giroux, É. (2021). Can populations be healthy? Perspectives from Georges Canguilhem and Geoffrey Rose. *History and Philosophy of the Life Sciences*, *43*(4), 111. https://doi.org/10.1007/s40656-021-00463-x

Goldberg, D.S. (2012). Social justice, health inequalities and methodological individualism in US health promotion. *Public Health Ethics*, *5*(2), 104–115. https://doi.org/10.1093/phe/phs013

Hancock, B.H. (2018). Michel Foucault and the problematics of power: Theorizing DTCA and medicalized subjectivity. *The Journal of Medicine and Philosophy*, *43*(4), 439–468. https://doi.org/10.1093/jmp/jhy010

Harvey, A. (2010). Genetic risks and healthy choices: Creating citizen-consumers of genetic services through empowerment and facilitation. *Sociology of Health & Illness*, *32*(3), 365–381. https://doi.org/10.1111/j.1467–9566.2009.01202.x

Jasanoff, S. (2015). Future imperfect. In S. Jasanoff & S.H-. Kim (Eds.), *Dreamscapes of modernity: Sociotechnical imaginaries and the fabrication of power* (pp. 1–33). The University of Chicago Press.
Jasanoff, S., & Kim, S.H-. (2009). Containing the atom: Sociotechnical imaginaries and nuclear regulation in the U.S. and South Korea. *Minerva*, *47*(2), 119–146. https://doi.org/10.1007/s11024-009-9124-4
Kierkegaard, S. (1980 [1849]). *The sickness unto death: A Christian psychological exposition for upbuilding and awakening* (H.V. Hong & E. H. Hong, trans.). Princeton University Press.
Laverack, G. (2017). The challenge of behaviour change and health promotion. *Challenges*, *8*(2), 25. https://doi.org/10.3390/challe8020025
Lewis, T. (2008). *Smart living: Lifestyle media and popular expertise.* Peter Lang Publishing.
Obama, B. (2007, March 23). Genomics and personalized medicine act of 2007. https://www.govtrack.us/congress/bills/110/s976/text
Parsons, T. (1951). *The social system.* Tavistock Publications.
Petersen, A. (2019). *Digital health and technological promise.* Routledge.
Philips, C.J. (2020). Precision medicine and its imprecise history. *Harvard Data Science Review*, 2(1), 1–10.
Pokorksa-Bocci, A., Stewart, A., Sagoo, G.S., Hall, A., Kroese, M., & Burton, H. (2014). 'Personalized medicine': What's in a name? *Personalized Medicine*, *11*(2), 197–210. https://doi.org/10.2217/pme.13.107
Prainsack, B. (2017). *Personalized medicine: Empowered patients in the 21st century?* New York University Press.
Puhl, R.M., & C.A. Heuer. (2009). The stigma of obesity: A review and update. *Obesity*, *17*(5), 941–996. https://doi.org/10.1038/oby.2008.636
Strand, R. (2022). The impact of a fantasy. In C. Beneduce & M. Bertolaso (Eds.), *Personalized medicine in the making: Philosophical perspectives from biology to healthcare* (pp. 311–324). Springer.
Tengland, P.A-. (2012). Behavior change or empowerment: On the ethics of health-promotion strategies. *Public Health Ethics*, *5*(2), 140–153. https://doi.org/10.1093/phe/phs022
Tengland, P.A-. (2016). Behavior change or empowerment: On the ethics of health-promotion goals. *Health Care Analysis*, *24*(1), 24–46. https://doi.org/10.1007/s10728-013-0265-0
The Precision Medicine Initiative. (2015). So what is precision medicine? https://obamawhitehouse.archives.gov/precision-medicine
Toro, J., Kiverstein, J., & Rietveld, E. (2020). The ecological-enactive model of disability: Why disability does not entail pathological embodiment. *Frontiers in Psychology*, *11*, 1162. https://doi.org/10.3389/fpsyg.2020.01162
Tutton, R. (2014). *Genomics and the reimagination of personalized medicine.* Ashgate Publishing.
Vogt, H., Hofmann, B., & Getz, L. (2016). The new holism: P4 systems medicine and the medicalization of health and life itself. *Medicine, Health Care and Philosophy*, *19*(2), 307–323. https://doi.org/10.1007/s11019-016-9683-8
World Health Organization. (2021). *Health Promotion Glossary of Terms 2021.* Geneva.

Epilogue

There is a lot in this book that has not been said. This concerns the way the framework relates to other philosophically inspired accounts of health, the distinction between the medical and the molecular gaze, and the intersubjective nature of healthy embodiment. In this epilogue, I will offer some starting points for connecting my phenomenological account of healthy embodiment to the above issues.

Relationality and Experiential Unity

One of the main implications of the approach to the healthy body developed in this book is that a body is not a rigid, stable, unmalleable object with a definite shape and clear boundaries, but instead is made up of relations. This relationality can be expressed with reference to the different aspects of the body: *Leib*, *Körper*, and *Body as Part of a Population*. None of these aspects exist independent of one another, but it is the relations between those aspects that determines how we experience our own body and its health status, as well as our relationship to the environment. Put differently, it is through these relations that the world that one inhabits is constituted, as is one's experience of being able to cope with the particular demands of this world.

What I have further emphasised throughout this book is that health importantly consists in one's capacity to be normative, and to not completely coincide with the norms being exercised upon one, such that the experience of health is irreducible to one of the aspects of one's body. In line with Canguilhem, health is understood as a way of coping with the demands of the environment that are continuously changing as a result of environmental irregularities, social norms and technoscientific developments. Sociotechnical imaginaries, such as that of personalised medicine, as well as technologies developed for health promotion and disease prevention, embody particular health norms and reshape the relations between the different aspects of one's body, thereby shaping healthy embodiment.

DOI: 10.4324/9781003602385-7

Since one's body is constituted by the relationships between its different aspects, these technologies and imaginaries make it that new bodies are constituted that exercise their normativity in novel ways.

At first sight, this approach to the experience of health that is grounded in the relational constitution of one's body resembles recent approaches that take health to be a particular assemblage. Such approaches similarly deny the existence of a more or less stable body that can function as a reference point and on which "health" can be predicated. There are, however, subtle but important differences between an "assemblage account of health" and the approach endorsed in this book. The key underlying difference is that my approach grants that the (healthy) body results from the particular relations between its different aspects but, in spite of this, still appears as an *experiential unity*. Let me further elaborate on this point by means of a brief comparative discussion.

Assemblage approaches to health typically take inspiration from the work of Gilles Deleuze. The English term "assemblage" is the translation of the French word "agencement", which can be translated as "a construction, an arrangement, or a layout" (Nail, 2017, p. 22). On Deleuze's account, everything is an assemblage; everything is made up of a particular arrangement of relations without a central core that organises those relations. In the absence of such a core, all arrangements are inherently unstable and lack any particular essence. Assemblages are made up of contingent interactions that grant temporary stability. Whether we speak about a human, a city, a desktop or a microphone, we speak about assemblages that are different because they happen to be made up of different relations, but not because of some a priori differences between them. As Deleuze emphasises, these assemblages are different as a result of what they can *do*, instead of what they *are* (Deleuze, 1992, p. 257 *op. cit.* Duff, 2014, p. 41).

The notion of assemblage has the advantage of acknowledging that humans do not have a specific place within the larger network that they are part of and are not considered loci of control or autonomous decision-making. This is why Law and Mol (2020, p. 64) have described the notion of assemblage as an "agency-decentring term", indicating that human beings are assemblages too and should not be understood as the centre from which activities of nonhumans are organised. Rather, the human being and the world that it inhabits result from contingent interactions that are constitutive of them but for which humans cannot be held solely responsible. These interactions range from biological and environmental demands to the sociopolitical norms that structure reality.

In *The Body Multiple*, Mol tries to cash out an assemblage understanding of reality in the context of medicine. In the book, she argues, through an ethnographic analysis of atherosclerosis, that the human body is not a singular thinking but takes shape differently in different contexts without it being possible to identify a stable core across these different contexts. This is why she speaks of the body multiple: what a body *is*, is dependent on the assemblages of which it is a part. The body with atherosclerosis at home watching television with a slight pain simply is a different thing than the body with atherosclerosis as examined by a general practitioner. And the body examined by a general practitioner is different from the body examined by a cardiologist or neurologist. For Mol, revealing the multiple ways in which the body is enacted serves to indicate that it is impossible to make bodies adhere to a singular standard of health or normality. The crux here is that the body is ontologically distinct when part of different assemblages, such that the knowledge of it cannot be assembled in one meta-assemblage that tells the final story about what the body with atherosclerosis really is. Showing multiplicity, then, contributes "to theorizing medicine's *ontological politics*: a politics that has to do with the way in which problems are framed, bodies are shaped, and lives are pushed into one shape or another" (Mol, 2002, p. viii).

While Mol's work is critical for understanding the different normativities that prevail in medical practice, she does not explicitly extend her work to the experience of healthy embodiment. Duff's *Assemblages of Health* (2014) explicitly draws from Deleuze's thought on assemblages to develop a new way of thinking about health. Duff's goal is to use assemblage theory to approach health "as a particular state of embodied subjectivity that is formed or produced in an assemblage of relations, affects and events" (Duff, 2014, p. xiii). Similarly to the approach taken in this book, Duff argues that a philosophical approach to health should "abandon the reified body of biomedicine, along with its ineluctable biology" (Duff, 2014, p. 6). He calls for a replacement of this body with an understanding of health in terms of studying "bodies in their posthuman assembling, in their becoming well or ill" (Duff, 2014, p. 6). The latter marks a very specific way of abandoning the reified body of medicine, as well as a replacement of what health should be attributed to: "health ought to be regarded as a property of the assemblage and not of any one individual body" (Duff, 2014, p. 35).

What, then, does it mean for health to be a property of an assemblage and what is the relationship between this understanding of health and the embodied experience of health? Answering these questions helps outline one key similarity and two major differences between an assemblage approach to health and the one outlined in this book. The similarity consists in that Duff's reading of Deleuze makes him conclude that "health cannot be said to pertain solely to a remote physiological entity" (Duff, 2014, p. 185) and that the "relational imbrication of bodies and milieus admits of no ontological distinction between the two" (Duff, 2014, p. 81).

This aligns with the basic phenomenological insight that health is not a property of the *Körper* or can be attributed to the *Körper* otherwise, but instead manifests in the "I can"; the ability to habitually transcend into a meaningful reality. And given that the experience of healthy embodiment results, in line with Canguilhem, from the ability to cope with a multiplicity of environments that are partly of human making, it is indeed fair to say that in a sense there is no clear-cut answer to the question of where the organism ends and the environment begins.

The reasons why the answer to this question is not clear-cut differ in the assemblage account of health. By taking the general category of life as a starting point, before it is being individualised and manifests in a concrete organismic form. It is life, then, that blurs the boundaries between the body and environment because it "is always distributed in and among a series of territories or milieus; a multiplicity or assemblage of forces rather than a singular, stable organismal form" (Duff, 2014, p. 73). Life, then, precedes its organismic or material instantiation. In this sense, the assemblage account differs from the one presented in this book; whereas it shares the ideas that health does not contain in maintaining organismic stability and that any organism lacks a particular blueprint with regard to how health can be realised, I take as a starting point that the experience of health minimally involves the *experience* of being distinct from the environment in which it manifests. The experience of non-indifference is a necessary condition for taking any kind of entity to be a living one; to merge completely with the environment such that any friction disappears is to become non-living. Put differently, the embodied experience of health minimally presupposes the experience of being different from other elements that are part of the assemblage in which one is integrated.

The second difference between Duff's assemblage account of health and the one developed in this book lies in the way the notion of health is conceptualised. He characterises health "as a discontinuous process of affective and relational becoming in which the quality of life is advanced in the provision of new affective sensitivities and new relational capacities" (Duff, 2014, p. xiii), and as a "differential process of becoming reasonable, strong and free, where freedom is understood not in some totalising way synonymous with a prevailing moral order, but rather as a specific moment of rupture or transformation in which something new emerges in an active expression of creativity and invention" (Duff, 2014, p. 17). Differentiation, then, becomes synonymous with having the power to act and an indication of having this power is to experience joy in the activities that one carries out (Duff, 2014, p. 83). I read these characterisations of health as referring to the capacity of exercising power[1] within a manifold of forces and finding joy when exercising this very capacity.

This characterisation echoes a Nietzschean view on health, which should not be too much of a surprise given Deleuze's extensive engagement with Nietzsche's work. Welsh endorses a similar Nietzschean view of health when describing it—pace phenomenological accounts—as an intense experience that is not necessarily hidden (2016, p. 348). It is intense events—such as illness and the overcoming of it—that give life meaning, and living through those events and having the power to incorporate them into existence is an indication of living a healthy life. The idiosyncrasy of these events and the specific ways in which one deals with them are manifestations of the subject's process of differentiation. They enable the subject to determine itself what constitutes health, as well as enables it to differentiate itself from prevailing health norms.

Whereas the account of health developed in this book aligns with the idea that health is not to be equated with the body being transparent in experience such that the subject is directed at what is external to it, it also finds the account of health as we find in Welsh's or Duff's work too demanding. In this sense, I side with Svenaeus' (2019) response to a Nietzschean critique of phenomenological accounts of health and illness. Svenaeus argues that indeed many intense events might give meaning to one's life and even contribute to leading a more authentic life, but that incorporating such events into an account of health is to mix up (the experience of) being healthy with other things, such as moral superiority and happiness (2019, p. 473). While such experiences might be certainly important and are indicators of one's quality of life (cf. Duff, 2014, p. xiii) and might make subjects more creative or inventive, they are in itself no markers of health when health is understood in Canguilhem's more minimal sense.

Beyond the Medical Gaze? Biomedicalisation and the Molecular Gaze

One of the key ideas behind developing a broader notion of health is that the medical gaze has changed shape, leading to an increasing normativisation of health by means of which acting healthy has become treated as a moral duty and that increasingly many phenomena of everyday life are filed under the category of health (e.g., Greco, 2004; Metzl, 2010). Rose, for instance, argues that "contemporary medical technologies do not seek merely to cure diseases once they have manifested themselves, but to control the vital processes of the body and mind. They are, I suggest, technologies of optimisation" (2007, p. 16). This, in turn, gives rise to what can be called a "good health imperative" (Welsh, 2022) as a result of which optimisation is taken as a moral duty that individuals themselves are to a large extent responsible for. This is because technoscientific breakthroughs in the life sciences and neurosciences give rise to the idea that increasingly many aspects of the body and mind can and should be controlled and should be integrated into the good health imperative. These changes, then, are understood as a break with earlier forms of medicalisation because the body as part of a population is construed differently and is made subject to different social norms.

To assess whether we should indeed speak of a break with earlier forms of medicine, it is necessary to establish if the body as part of a population has indeed changed shape through the development from a clinical gaze into what can be called a more-than-clinical gaze. For Rose, whereas the principal objects of the clinical gaze were illness and disease and the underlying science was pathology, the principal object of the molecular gaze is health and its underlying science is molecular biology. The clinical gaze, as described in Foucault, is, on Rose's account, grounded in the activity of doctors who directly relate to patients, interpret their visible symptoms and link those to an underlying pathology. Patients and their environment, then, become objects of medical inquiry and intervention when attempting to create a relationship between them that cures or prevents identifiable pathologies. This, for Rose, is a very specific style of biopolitics that is left behind in the age of the molecular sciences (Rose, 2007, pp. 11–12). These sciences give rise to a different problematisation of health in which it is ingrained in an engineering metaphor of life as something that can and should be controlled by its carrier. Rather than constituting an environment that does not contribute to the death or deterioration of the organism, medicine starts to revolve around the development and promotion of specific regimes of the self in which health itself becomes an object of management for which individuals have become responsible.

Similar to Rose, Clarke and colleagues (2003, 2010) notice a shift from medicalisation to *biomedicalisation* that accompanies a shift from the clinical to the molecular gaze. This shift is characterised by an increasing convergence of the practice of medicine and the life sciences, such as molecular biology, and is clearly visible in sociotechnical imaginaries like personalised medicine. As a result of this convergence, people are generally taken to be continuously at risk of becoming unhealthy, leading up to an individualised good health imperative. This is further fuelled by the increasing presence of medical information that is distributed through all kinds of popular media channels. Since people are, in principle, able to take note of this information, they are held responsible for collecting this information, interpreting it and integrating it into their own lives. In addition, medicine is no longer integrally tied to state funding but has become increasingly corporatised and privatised, which makes it impossible to tie medicalisation to a single source or the protection of the destiny of a particular nation as Foucault seems to suggest (Clarke & Shim, 2011). The spread of medical information, the nature of medical interventions, as well as the responsibility of citizens also tie in with financial interests of companies. Health, then, has become a form of capital.

Together, these ideas suggest that since the molecular gaze essentially opens up the living inside of the human body, death is no longer the starting point of medicalisation, and that medicalisation no longer originates from the interests of nation-states but no longer a central location. This results in a shift from understanding of medicine in terms of the metaphor of the clinic to one revolving around what Rose has termed the *politics of life itself*. The main results of this shift are that life itself has become an object of governmental concern that is in need of continuous self-management, that the way this management should take place is partly guided by commercial interests, and that increasingly many aspects of one's body appear as governable. A notable example here is the appearance of the brain as an object of government due to developments in the neurosciences (Rose & Abi-Rached, 2013). A new form of subjectivity emerges due to the politics of life itself, in which health explicitly comes to the fore as something that the subject is responsible for and which becomes part of the experiential structure through which the subject understands itself and the world around it.

The framework developed in this book is sympathetic to the above ideas: I am not denying that contemporary medicine indeed takes health—instead of illness or disease—to be its primary object, neither that it tends to make people increasingly responsible for their own health, nor that medicine has become increasingly intertwined with commercial interests that result in a commodification of health. What I am questioning is the extent to which this change—or transformation—accompanies a change in the embodied experience of health such that it no longer can be captured in terms of the relationship(s) between *Leib*, *Körper*, and body as part of a population.

In response to the work of Clarke and colleagues, Conrad (2005) argues that the identified changes are changes in degree and not indicative of a fundamental shift. He suggests that the engines that drive medicalisation have changed without altering the basis of medicalisation itself. Whereas for a long time doctors were the main drivers of medicalisation, currently, they have been become more marginal in this respect and have been replaced by commercial actors and patient care organisations. Additionally, technologies have become increasingly important in medicalising phenomena. As should be clear from the phenomenological analysis of human-technology relations in the context of healthcare and my characterisation of personalised medicine as a sociotechnical imaginary that shapes embodied subjectivity, these changing drivers can be incorporated into the framework developed in this book: it provides a meta-explanation of how the developments sketched by Rose and Clarke et al. shape the embodied experience of health by laying bare how these changes affect the relations between the different aspects of our body.

Take the example of personalised medicine: it can be characterised as a particular problematisation of health that forefronts, on the one hand, that diagnostics and treatment should be more tailor-made to individuals and their biological make-up, whereas, on the other hand, it also suggest that health is largely dependent on the lifestyles of individuals and hence partly falls within the individual's domain of control. Both forms of problematisation are dependent on technologies that either increase the diagnostic and therapeutic effectiveness of medical professionals or contribute to making relevant health parameters more visible to individuals such that they can allegedly exercise (more) control over them.

The ideal of personalising medicine presupposes the existence of a particular kind of population, such that certain standards of normality can be determined. Both diagnostic accuracy and the notion of a healthy lifestyle assume that individuals are part of a larger population that develops in relation to some standard of normality. Even if many developments in personalised medicine no longer work with a notion of population as tied to the sole interest of maintaining the number of inhabitants of a nation-state, the notion of population has not been dissolved but rather has become scattered. One can be part of many different populations, which—as I have argued—creates a possibility of counter-conduct: by opposing the idea that, for instance a certain age group is a relevant population to be part of, one can challenge the demands of personalised medicine.

The condition of possibility for this or alternative forms of counter-conduct is precisely that the emergence of the imaginary of personalised medicine reshapes the relational structure of *Leib*, *Körper*, and *Body as Part of a Population*. It involves the ideal of a deliberate thematisation of health as an object of experience such that—through the emergence of novel processes of normalisation—the *Körper* is constituted differently as a carrier of all kinds of medical risks that individuals can and might want to avoid. This, in turn, shapes the "I can", the intentional relation of the individual to the world. It shapes the projects that individuals wish to carry out, the things that stand out as objects of concern, as well as one's relation to one's own body. This shift is significant because it results in an increasing number of situations in which health is no longer an experience of bodily transparency but becomes a thematic on its own. However, and this is why I would be hesitant to speak of a radical break with the earlier clinical gaze, the same aspects of the body remain to condition what can be experienced as healthy even when one of those aspects starts appearing as more central than the other. This also explains why the process of medicalisation and its normative inscribing are successful: since we literally *are* bodies as part of a population, inscriptions on a population inevitably become part of our (self-)experience.

Normality and Intersubjectivity

Since the *Body as Part of a Population* is key to the experience of health, standards of normality are key to understanding healthy embodiment. And since standards of normality are irreducible to particular individuals, the experience of health always takes shape to a certain extent in one's relationship with others. As a result, health is intersubjectively constituted in the relationship(s) between different bodies. Throughout this book, I have not paid specific attention to the phenomenon of intersubjectivity in the context of health precisely because I think that it can be to a large extent explained by how institutionalised norms become part of embodied experience through a power dynamics that is exemplified in Foucault's work.

However, at this point, it is apt to devote a few words to explicate why and how health is never an individual experience but presupposes what Merleau-Ponty (1968) in the *Visible and the Invisible* has called *intercorporeity*: to exist as an embodied being necessarily entails to be intertwined with other embodied beings, such that our perceptions and experiences are constituted in virtue of this intertwinement and are therefore to a certain extent shared. This is also why I can experience that somebody else feels unhealthy and the other way around, why I can evaluate (for better or worse) someone else's lifestyle in terms of certain health parameters and hold that others are to a certain extent responsible for their own health. For Merleau-Ponty, intercorporeity is always dynamic as my own body and the body of others are subject to change as a result of particular habitual patterns or technological developments (de Boer & Verbeek, 2022), which also leads to changing relations between bodies and hence to changing experiences of health. Intercorporeity is a condition of possibility for entering a shared world in which communication and meaningful interactions with others are possible, as well as shaping my own embodied intentionality (Moran, 2017). In recognising others as living embodied beings and in being recognised as a lived embodied being by others, it becomes possible to inhabit a meaningful environment that I am familiar with. To put it in Merleau-Ponty's terms, intercorporeity is constitutive of the "I can".

At the same time, as has been aptly recognised by many key thinkers in the phenomenological tradition such as Husserl, Heidegger and Merleau-Ponty, the shared world that we inhabit also constitutes embodiment passively. After all, to exist is to be thrown into a world that is already stabilised and has an already existing structure of signification that is materialised in institutions, norms and technological artefacts. And given an increasing tendency to medicalise more aspects of our everyday lives, medical norms and institutions, as well as medical technologies, play an important role in the passive constitution of embodiment. It is, of course for precisely this reason that Foucault's analyses of power have figured so prominently in this book: they form the basis of an embodied orientation to the normal from which the experience of oneself and others can deviate.

Embodied forms of normalisation feed back into the unreflective structure of experience but are neither static nor universal. For instance, Mauss's (1973 [1936]) discussions of how different generations are taught how to swim differently show that particular norms are tacitly integrated into one's structure of embodiment. And similarly, Young's (1980) famous description of how girls embody a particular movement style while throwing a ball shows how particular norms (e.g., this is the normal way of swimming!, it is risky for girls to practice baseball) passively constitute movement patterns and shape how the world is experienced. It is by means of these norms that a shared world becomes possible and meaningful interaction with others can take place; they form the basis for distinguishing between what is familiar and what is deviant, and between what is correct and what is incorrect.

Wehrle (2015, 2016) notes that because of the inevitable presence of normalisation, our world is ambiguous in that it provides us with both opportunities for positive interactions and violent constraints. She argues that a combination of a Foucauldian and a phenomenological approach is needed for understanding embodied normality. On the one hand, the Foucauldian tradition has emphasised the process of what she calls *violent normalisation* by means of which disciplinary norms are inscribed into the body and shape embodied experiences. On the other hand, the phenomenological tradition has primarily conceptualised embodiment in terms of a productive and operative "I can" that enables people to meaningfully interact with the environment through the development of particular habits. Her key point is that the habits that people develop do not solely originate from the individual's idiosyncratic history and preferences but are also the result of the norms that are present in a shared intersubjective world.

The importance of normality in phenomenology is a way to take very seriously the idea that to exist is to be in a particular situation: existence is situatedness (Wehrle, 2021). And to be situated implies to be inevitably confronted with a cultural, material, technoscientific and intersubjective reality that partly determines what is normal. It is against this background, in line with what I earlier wrote about Canguilhem in chapter 4, that the individual exercises their own normativity. Hence, the presence of particular medical institutions, technologies used to manage healthcare, or socio-technical imaginaries surrounding medicine instantiate particular forms of normality that become part of the embodied experience of health. These norms, as I have tried to show throughout the book, are pervasive and influential. This is, for instance, visible in how increasingly many people nowadays tend to understand health as an object that can be visualised and manipulated. It is this visibility that currently is the standard for entering the intersubjective world of being healthy and which is the condition of possibility for both concerted actions to realise particular health goals, and the stigmatisation of others that allegedly do not conform to one's own embodied normativity.

Albeit brief, this discussion suggests that intersubjectivity is not foreign to my account of healthy embodiment: the experience of normality is an intersubjective experience of health. This view on intersubjectivity is the direct result of integrating a Foucauldian approach into phenomenology. I concede that this approach to intersubjectivity is not exhaustive and does not directly address how the experience of health, for instance results from the explicit experience of being perceived by other beings, nor outlines in detail how interactions with particular individuals or groups give rise to particular forms of healthy embodiment. What it does indicate, however, is that the individuals one interacts with and is perceived by, as well as the groups that one is part of or is excluded from, are also the result of the presence of an embodied normality that structures the zero-point of orientation from which other things appear as relevant.

I started this book by problematising Gadamer's famous idea that health remains inevitably enigmatic. Health's transparency is only one way in which it can be integrated into embodiment. In this case, the constitution of healthy embodiment is such that health is experienced mainly interpreted in terms of the *Leib*. However, this interpretation is not a phenomenological or experiential given but instead a particular manifestation of the relationship between *Leib*, *Körper*, and the *Body as Part of a Population*. Or, put differently, it is only a particular way of embodying health norms. Whereas Canguilhem was still able to write in *The Normal and the Pathological* that only when "I am unwell, people want to know how and why; they wonder or ask me whether I am registered with social security" (Canguilhem, 2012, p. 51), the social norms around health have changed since the publication of the book in 1943. This has given rise to a different manifestation of healthy embodiment in which the *Body as Part of a Population* becomes the main axis along which health is experienced. Be it the shift towards personalised medicine, the increasing popularity of health-related technologies developed by medical institutions and companies alike, the popularity of fitness programmes advertised on social media or in workplaces, health is explicitly present as an observable standard that shapes how we interpreting ourselves, shapes how we are interpreted by others, as well as shapes how we interpret other people. The presence of this standard marks a different way of embodying normality than assumed in the remarks by Gadamer and Canguilhem.

Throughout this book, I have been largely neutral—or agnostic—about the desirability of explicitly thematising health such that it becomes increasingly present as an object of experience. Of course, the Foucauldian analysis of the power of medical institutions, as well as the focus on medicalisation, implicitly points to a concern—powerfully put on the agenda by Illich—about the extent to which our (self-)experience is guided by external and contingent medical norms. These perspectives suggest that there is a tipping point after which the presence of medicine goes at the expense of people's capacity to make autonomous decisions when it comes to life's inevitable sufferings. I hope that this book can contribute to an ongoing critical discussion of the ways in which medical norms shape our lives. This requires to acknowledge that there is no safe authentic space that is not contiminated by medical norms and to which we can return.

Note

1 Following Deleuze (and Foucault for that matter), Duff warns not to understand notions like "power" or "strength" in terms of a force that one actor exerts over another actor (2014, p. 162). Rather, power consists in being able to be affected by its numerous relations to other bodies and the capacity to organise oneself in relation to those affects.

References

Canguilhem, G. (2012). *Writings on medicine* (S. Geroulanos & T. Meyers, trans.). Fordham University Press.

Clarke, A.E., & Shim, J.K. (2011). Medicalization and biomedicalization revisited: Technoscience and transformations of health, illness and American medicine. In B.A. Pescosolido, J.K. Martin, J.D. McLeod, & A. Rogers (Eds.), *Handbook of the sociology of health, illness, and healing* (pp. 173–200). Springer.

Clarke, A.E., Shim, J.K., Mamo, L., Ruth Fosket, J., & Fishman, J.R. (2003). Biomedicalization: Technoscientific transformations of health, illness, and U.S. Biomedicine. *American Sociological Review*, *68*(2), 161–194. https://doi.org/10.2307/1519765

Clarke, A.E., Shim, J.K., Mamo, L., Ruth Fosket, J., & Fishman, J.R. (2010). Biomedicalization: A theoretical and substantive introduction. In A.E. Clarke, J.K. Shim, L. Mamo, J. Ruth Fosket, & J.R. Fishman (Eds.), *Biomedicalization: Technoscience, health, and illness in the U.S.* (pp. 1–44). Duke University Press.

Conrad, P. (2005). The shifting engines of medicalization. *Journal of Health and Social Behavior*, *46*(1), 3–14. https://doi.org/10.1177/002214650504600102

de Boer, B., & Verbeek, P.P-. (2022). Living in the flesh: Technologically mediated chiasmic relationships (in times of a pandemic). *Human Studies*, *45*, 189–208. https://doi.org/10.1007/s10746-022-09625-7

Deleuze, G. (1992). Postscript on the societies of control. *October*, *59*, 3–7.

Duff, C. (2014). *Assemblages of health: Deleuze's empiricism and the ethology of life*. Springer.

Greco, M. (2004). The politics of indeterminacy and the right to health. *Theory, Culture & Society*, *21*(6), 1–22. https://doi.org/10.1177/0263276404047413

Law, J., & Mol, A. (2020). Words to think with: An introduction. *The Sociological Review Monographs*, *68*(2), 263–282. https://doi.org/10.1177/0038026120905452

Mauss, M. (1973 [1936]). Techniques of the body. *Economy & Society*, *2*(1), 70–88.

Merleau-Ponty, M. (1968). *The visible and the invisible* (A. Lingis, trans.). Northwestern University Press.

Metzl, J.M. (2010). Why "against health"?. In J.M. Metzl & A. Kirkland (Eds.), *Against health: How health became the new morality* (pp. 1–13). New York University Press.

Mol, A. (2002). *The body multiple: Ontology in medical practice*. Duke University Press.

Moran, D. (2017). Intercorporeality and intersubjectivity: A phenomenological exploration of embodiment. In C. Durt, T. Fuchs, & C. Tewes (Eds.), *Embodiment, enaction, and culture: Investigating the constitution of the shared world* (pp. 25–46). The MIT Press.

Nail, T. (2017). What is an assemblage? *SubStance*, *46*(1), 21–37. https://doi.org/10.1353/sub.2017.001

Rose, N. (2007). *The politics of life itself: Biomedicine, power, and subjectivity in the twenty-first century*. Princeton University Press.

Rose, N., & Abi-Rached, J.M. (2013). *Neuro: The new brain sciences and the management of the mind*. Princeton University Press.

Svenaeus, F. (2019). A defense of the phenomenological account of health and illness. *Journal of Medicine and Philosophy*, *44*(4), 459–478. https://doi.org/10.1093/jmp/jhz013

Wehrle, M. (2015). Normality and normativity in experience. In M. Doyon & T. Breyer (Eds.), *Normativity in perception* (pp. 128–139). Palgrave MacMillan.

Wehrle, M. (2016). Normative embodiment. The role of the body in Foucault's genealogy. A phenomenological re-reading. *Journal of the British Society for Phenomenology*, *47*(1), 56–71. https://doi.org/10.1080/00071773.2015.1105645

Wehrle, M. (2021). Situating normality: The interrelation of lived and represented reality. *Chiasmi International*, *23*, 99–119. https://doi.org/10.5840/chiasmi20212322

Welsh, T. (2016). Many healths: Nietzsche and phenomenologies of illness. *Frontiers of Philosophy in China*, *11*(3), 338–357. https://doi.org/10.3868/s030-005-016-0026-3

Welsh, T. (2022). *Feminist existentialism, biopolitics, and critical phenomenology in a time of bad health*. Routledge.

Young, I.M. (1980). Throwing like a girl: A phenomenology of feminine body comportment motility and spatiality. *Human Studies*, *3*(2), 137–156.

Index

For Product Safety Concerns and Information please contact our EU
representative GPSR@taylorandfrancis.com
Taylor & Francis Verlag GmbH, Kaufingerstraße 24, 80331 München, Germany

www.ingramcontent.com/pod-product-compliance
Ingram Content Group UK Ltd.
Pitfield, Milton Keynes, MK11 3LW, UK
UKHW022355190926
475702UK00015B/2308
* 9 7 8 1 0 3 2 9 9 1 1 3 9 *